WORRIED SICK
Our Troubled Quest for Wellness

WORRIED SICK
Our Troubled Quest for Wellness

ARTHUR J. BARSKY, M.D.

LITTLE, BROWN AND COMPANY
BOSTON   TORONTO

FIRST EDITION

Library of Congress Cataloging-in-Publication Data

Barsky, Arthur J.
  Worried sick.

  Bibliography: p.
  Includes index.
  1. Health behavior—United States.   2. Sick—
United States—Psychology.   I. Title.
RA445.B38   1988   613'.01'9   87-32508
ISBN 0-316-08255-4

10   9   8   7   6   5   4   3   2   1

Designed by Robert G. Lowe

RRD VA

Published simultaneously in Canada
by Little, Brown & Company (Canada) Limited

PRINTED IN THE UNITED STATES OF AMERICA

To my father

Contents

Preface

AT THE AGE of forty-four, I find I'm every bit as concerned about my health as the next person. I try hard to run three times a week, I'm fighting (none too successfully) to keep my weight from creeping up, and I pester my children not to salt their food. I have my own doctor and I see him regularly for checkups. I believe that these things are beneficial, so I do them myself, and as a doctor I prescribe them for others. Although in portions of this book I am critical of some contemporary attitudes about health, I do not mean to deride the impetus toward taking better care of ourselves, or to impugn the value of most of what we're doing along those lines.

I just don't want my health concerns to take over my life, and I've noticed that health consciousness has a way of getting out of hand and getting blown out of proportion. Looking after your health may be one of those pursuits it is possible to try too hard at, so that the undertaking becomes unnecessarily unpleasant, or perhaps even compromises its success. Earlier today, I took my children swimming at a nearby lake. At ten minutes before each hour, a burly lifeguard climbed a tower at the edge of the beach and announced over the loudspeaker, "Could I have your attention? This is *not* an emergency; we're going to have a routine beach check. Will all swimmers please leave the water and return to their spots on the beach. If anyone you are with fails to join your party, please let us know immediately." Ten uneventful minutes later, when we are allowed back in the water, the lifeguards resume their sentry duty, policing the children who climb onto the dock and warning others of the hazards of various water games. Kids must be taught proper water safety, and they must learn to respect the all-too-real dangers of swimming and diving. Indeed, a child drowned at this very lake only two summers ago. But as we left, I realized that trying so hard to make things safe had taken some of the fun out of them—it all felt so restricted and inhibited, so supervised and policed. We need to be careful lest something similar happen to us as we cope with all of the threats there are to health.

The idea for this book grew out of my clinical work at the Massachusetts General Hospital, where I have worked for the last fourteen years. I was treating patients who had serious medical illnesses, trying to help them deal with their predicaments and make the most of what they had left, and to facilitate their search for meaning and gratification in life despite their suffering and illness. It was astonishing how different people's experiences were. Some were cheerful and peaceful and considerate of others while in the midst of the most devastating illnesses. Others felt empty, angry, and demoralized. How sick they felt often seemed unrelated to how sick we as doctors thought they were. It was their distress, their struggles, and their successes that prodded me into thinking about the questions in this book more deeply. I should also add here that, although I've used their stories throughout the book, in all cases I have altered the particulars to protect the anonymity of my patients.

Intrigued by this enormous individual variation in experiencing disease, I began a series of clinical research projects at Harvard Medical School in which I examined the psychological characteristics of people who coped unusually well with very serious illnesses and contrasted them with people who suffered unduly with minor ailments. I also began discussing these questions with my colleagues and with the medical students and interns and residents whom I regularly taught.

At about the same time, I began to be struck by how highly health conscious our whole society seemed to be getting. I didn't really leave my work behind when I went home at night because I encountered the same concerns and images and phrases in the world outside the hospital: the social conversation at parties turned more to health than to politics; medical reports were all over the newspapers and the nightly news; joggers seemed to be out at every hour of the day and night; my nonmedical friends began acquiring their own copies of the *Physicians' Desk Reference;* when we dined out, everyone got salads and no one ordered meat. There seemed to be parallels between the way some of my patients (especially the growing number of worried but basically healthy patients) felt about their own health, and the way health was regarded as a topic of general interest outside the world of medicine. Could we learn something about ourselves and our society by comparing and contrasting these public and private psychologies of health?

What led me into this exploration, then, helps to explain the organization of the book. The chapters fall into three sections. Chapters 1 through 4 explore the private psychology of health; they discuss how people perceive their bodies and think about their health. The basic point here is that how healthy you feel depends in large measure upon your psychological state and your situation in life and only partly reflects your objective health status. Chapters 5 through 8 present a kind of public psychology of health; they are an examination of what we as a society are doing and saying and thinking. Although our collective health status is very high, we are a society plagued by a sense of dis-ease and malaise and a seemingly constant need for medical care. Chapters 9 and 10 make up a third section, one that draws out some principles about health perception and then suggests how we might optimize our feelings of good health and physical well-being. The point is that the pursuit of health can be paradoxical. Secure physical well-being and self-confident vitality grow out of an acceptance of our frailties and our limits and our mortality as much as they result from our trying to cure every affliction, to evade every disease, and to relieve every symptom.

This book is written for people who find that health is more and more on their minds, and for people who want to look after themselves without it becoming too burdensome and worrisome. It is also written for those observers of the contemporary American scene who notice the growing health boom and wonder what it is all about, why it is occurring, and where it may lead.

I am a physician, not a journalist or a sociologist or a historian, all of whom might be better equipped to tackle this topic. Thus I undertook it with trepidation and a sense of humility. In addition, the topic is so broad and so immediate that it is rather like a fish trying to study the water he is swimming in. This book must be taken in that spirit—as tentative rather than definitive, as much an attempt to raise certain questions as to answer them. I've done my best to be accurate and careful, but the topic is so extensive and the "hard facts" so scanty that there is much room for interpretation. What I offer are possibilities as much as facts, suggestions as much as conclusions.

Acknowledgments

I AM INDEBTED to many people, in many ways. As is the case, I imagine, with any project that is really worth attempting, this book turned out to be far more challenging than I ever imagined it would be, and I could not have brought it even to this meager state without the help of so many.

Many of my colleagues provided thoughtful consideration over a prolonged period, in the spirit of intellectual exchange, even when they didn't necessarily endorse my thinking or my viewpoint. Heartfelt thanks go to Laurence R. Tancredi, M.D., Thomas P. Hackett, M.D., John D. Stoeckle, M.D., Gerald L. Klerman, M.D., Leon Eisenberg, M.D., John D. Goodson, M.D., and Jonathan F. Borus, M.D. Others met with me and shared the benefits of their reflections and their scholarship: Paul Starr, Ph.D., Arnold S. Relman, M.D., Irving K. Zola, Ph.D., Perry London, Ph.D., Renée C. Fox, Ph.D., James E. Groves, M.D., Arthur M. Kleinman, M.D., Christopher D. Gordon, M.D., and Edith Geringer, M.D.

Any number of friends were generous and patient enough to spend time and energy wending their way through earlier versions of the manuscript, which were even more ponderous and cumbersome than this one. Their assistance has been enormously important to me. I especially wish to thank Ken Sawyer, Jerry Mitchell, Barry Zitin, Fred Kahn, Dan Lederer, and Lee Lockwood.

I am equally indebted to those who worked with me in a professional capacity. Bill Phillips, an old friend who was also my editor, had a major role in this project. His clear vision of what this book should be like, and his calm persistence and guidance in getting it there were critical. Anne Conway made creative suggestions, did thoughtful and meticulous research, and constructed the historical vignette in chapter 1. Debbie Roth's and Peggy Freudenthal's editing was superb. Carla White and Kathy Latham also helped at many stages in the preparation of the manuscript.

My family not only tolerated my efforts, they nourished them. My son, Timothy, kept me company; my daughter Amy kept me thinking and questioning; and my daughter Emily always cheered me up. My wife, Susan, supported me in many ways through this whole enterprise. And Hannah Barsky, my mother, offered the breadth of her amazing intellect, as well as information that I could have found nowhere else.

And last, I am profoundly thankful to my patients. They have privileged me by sharing their most heartfelt experiences. They have talked about what matters most to them, and they have spoken honestly about themselves and their lives. It is in admiring their strengths and appreciating their struggles that I gained the insights presented here.

I thank you all.

WORRIED SICK
Our Troubled Quest for Wellness

CHAPTER 1

Doing Better and Feeling Worse

Frank Carson's Headaches

FRANKLIN CARSON'S ALARM CLOCK goes off as usual, but this morning it sounds like an ambulance siren. He is instantly jolted awake, his heart pounding, his mouth dry, his pillow damp with sweat: this is the day Frank has the appointment to see his doctor, and he fears he has developed a brain tumor. At thirty-seven, a market analyst for a computer firm, he has been married for eleven years. He and his wife, Barbara, have a nine-year-old daughter and are expecting their second child in three months. Frank has always been healthy; he seemed almost immune to colds and the flu, and he can't remember the last time he missed work because he didn't feel well. But a month ago, he developed dull, throbbing headaches that have steadily worsened. Then he felt faint several times after standing up suddenly. In the last two weeks, his vision seemed awfully blurry when he read fine print. Frank developed nausea late last week, and then he remembered how his mother had suffered with nausea when she was dying of a brain tumor. He had wondered in the past if brain cancer could be inherited, but he had never dared to ask anyone. Three days ago, terrified, he called his doctor for an appointment.

Chapter title from an article by Wildavsky, A. "Doing better and feeling worse: The political pathology of health policy." *Daedalus* 106 (1977): 105.

Rationally, Frank keeps telling himself that it's not anything serious; these must just be tension headaches from the stress he is under at work. But he can't seem to reassure himself that it's not something far more serious. For an instant, before he gets out of bed this morning, he imagines himself unable to get up, bald from cancer chemotherapy, and emaciated. He drives the image from his mind as he heads for the bathroom. Stepping on the scale, he compares this morning's weight with yesterday's. No matter what the numbers say, in the mirror he can still detect a sagging under his jaw, which betrays the advance of middle age. He turns up the shower with the pulsating head designed to improve muscle tone and blood flow, which he bought when he noticed a while back that his body was losing its tautness and firm tone. He shampoos with a special dandruff shampoo containing "medicinal ingredients" to correct "weakened" hair, and then "join[s] the crusade for healthy teeth and gums" (as the ad says) with Dentagard toothpaste.

Breakfast is on the kitchen table downstairs: decaffeinated coffee with a nondairy creamer, a high-fiber cereal, and vitamin pills. Frank loves eggs and bacon, but he stopped eating them to cut down on saturated fats. Feeling especially vulnerable this morning, he sneaks one of his daughter's calcium supplements for good measure. His eye is caught by some old mail lying in a sunny spot on the kitchen windowsill. It includes the usual avalanche of solicitations from societies to combat multiple sclerosis, muscular dystrophy, cystic fibrosis, and the rest. On his way out the back door, he notes that Barbara has stuck a newspaper clipping on the refrigerator door detailing the risks of alcohol and medications upon the developing fetus.

Time for the morning commute into New York City. He tries to concentrate on an upcoming marketing campaign, but soon the car radio distracts him with a "Report on Medicine" discussing the risk of contracting AIDS through casual contact; Frank is relieved since it sounds as if the chances are pretty low if you're not in a high-risk group—thank God he's never had a blood transfusion. Then there is an advertisement for Moisture Drops eyedrops, assuring him of the necessity for relief from "moisture-poor eyes." The world news at 8:00 includes an update on the status of the latest mechanical-heart recipient. Later, the station's financial reporter discusses the ins and outs of several new prepaid health-insurance plans. Finally, just as Frank pulls into the garage beneath his office building, there is a special report on the dangers of the summer sun as a cause of skin cancer: "If you're fair skinned, you're fair game for cancer." He practically lived on the beach for several summers as a teenager . . . can malignant skin cancers spread to the brain?

At work, Frank is called upon to make a brief presentation at a staff meeting. Several vice-presidents are present and he feels a great deal of pressure to do well. He feels his heart skip a beat, and he is flooded momentarily with terror: heart attack! He recalls that a physician who once examined him for an insurance physical had noted offhandedly that he had a heart murmur. But as Frank begins his presentation, his concern ebbs. Later on, pleased because his talk went well, he treats himself to a small self-indulgence: a stick of (sugarless) gum, more acceptable since its advertising claims that it doubles as a tooth cleanser.

He enjoys lunch with several old friends at a crowded local restaurant chosen for its excellent salad bar. The conversation centers on exercise regimens, jogging injuries, and the importance of dietary fiber. Three of the four people at the table have yogurt for dessert.

In the afternoon, already anxious about the imminent appointment with his doctor, Frank is handed a special project with a very tight deadline, and another of those headaches starts. Well, then, this proves it. The headaches must be due to stress after all—just his body's signal that he is pushing himself too hard, that he must learn to relax. Just before he leaves for his doctor's office, a memo crosses his desk announcing the opening of the company's "wellness" facility for employees that includes a gym, nutrition counseling, and a stress-reduction course. He vows to redouble his efforts to take better care of his precious health.

Twenty minutes with his physician, a thorough history, and a physical examination bring the verdict: "Frank, I don't see anything to make me suspect anything more serious than tension headaches. Just to be absolutely sure, I want to get a couple of tests while you're here. But what you describe is pretty classic. Obviously, if things change, if you get any new symptoms, you need to give me a call." Frank is overwhelmed with gratitude, profoundly thankful. It is as if he has been given another chance in life, as if the slate has been wiped clean. Now he can relinquish any thoughts of a grief-stricken widow and a fatherless nine-year-old. He can't wait to get home and tell Barbara; he'd been so frightened in the last few days that he had not discussed things with her at all.

An enormous weight has been lifted from Frank's shoulders. He feels full of energy, and when he arrives home, there is still time to jog his usual two-mile route. After the family dinner (broiled chicken and raw vegetables), Barbara leaves for her weekly childbirth class. Frank picks up the newspaper, discovers a special Health and Medicine section, and reads a long article by a television star whose father is dying from Alzheimer's disease.

Finally, after weighing himself again, flossing his teeth, and checking his resting pulse, he goes to bed. As he drifts off to sleep, he hears his pulse throbbing in his ear as it rests on the pillow, and though he received a clean bill of health only eight hours ago, he makes a mental note to remember to report this latest symptom to his doctor when he sees him next.

Being Well and Well-Being

Frank's health is crucial to him. He devotes a great deal of time and energy and money to taking good care of himself. "Wellness" is a quite conscious goal that he tries to achieve by adopting a healthy lifestyle. If he watches his weight and stays in shape, if he reduces stress and remembers to "buckle up," if he resists the temptations of chocolate and roast beef, if he sees his doctor "early and often," then surely he will reach the goal of "wellness."

And Frank is in fact completely healthy: his skin is young looking, his waist trim, his vision sharp. His electrocardiogram is normal, and his cholesterol level is low. Yet Frank doesn't *feel* healthy. He is troubled by symptoms, he worries about his health, he feels in need of medical care. A normal physical exam and a normal blood count don't allay a sense of dis-ease. In short, Frank can't enjoy the good health he does have.

There is something elusive, even counterproductive, about his quest for health: the more Frank consciously tries to be well, the less well-being he experiences. Running ten miles a week doesn't prevent him from worrying whether that mole on his shoulder has recently enlarged. Making sure that his family doesn't have any aluminum cooking pots doesn't quell the suspicion that a forgotten phone number is the first sign of Alzheimer's disease. The harder he tries to lose weight, the more dissatisfied he is with any hint of a spare tire around his middle; the more he tries to stave off the signs of aging, the more upsetting his thinning hair becomes. The more carefully he scrutinizes his body for ailments, the more things he finds wrong. The more new diseases he learns about in the newspapers, the more things he has to worry about—what could go wrong, what might go wrong, what has already, silently, gone wrong.

In Sickness and in Health

Frank is paradigmatic of contemporary America. Like him, our society devotes enormous human and economic resources to studying the body, staying healthy, and treating disease. And like Frank, we are a remarkably healthy society. But in spite of our success, there is a pervasive cultural atmosphere of dis-ease. Our sense of physical well-being has not kept pace with the improvements in our collective health status. The ability to appreciate our good health, a secure feeling of physical well-being and confident vigor, eludes us.

We are a society in headlong pursuit of health and medical care. As Frank's story illustrates, "wellness" has become a conscious goal, health something deliberately and consciously sought after. Good health, seen as an end in itself and not just as a means to other personal goals, has become an imperative, a sort of supervalue. It symbolizes personal achievement, self-esteem, and willpower. Every aspect of the body and of daily life is minutely scrutinized for its health implications and consequences, because we firmly believe that each individual has the power to control his health and thus to determine his own medical destiny. Through hard work and sustained effort, we seek to immunize ourselves against disease, conquer life's everyday ailments, and evade the physical decline of aging. Thus everything seems either healthful or harmful, and life becomes a series of prescribed and proscribed behaviors. Personal habits, diet, leisure activities are all modified to conform to the orthodoxy of the healthy lifestyle, as if there were one way of life that could assure us of complete and endless health.

The signs of this heightened health consciousness are all around us. Swimming pools, tracks, and weight rooms are jammed, and exercise is supposed to be the route to salvation here on earth. We are so preoccupied with nutrition that everything is either an elixir or a poison, and dieting has become the national pastime. Even people of perfectly normal size feel obese, and almost everyone has become a devotee of fish or pasta or calcium. Television, radio, the newspapers, and magazines are filled with medical advice and warnings about health. We are deluged with products and services to make us fit, keep us young, stave off disease, expunge every complaint. With each passing month, a different, usually horrible, disease achieves special notoriety (osteoporosis, sudden infant death syndrome, Alzheimer's disease, and, of course, AIDS). Health is being manufactured and marketed on a grand scale, and a medical-industrial complex is emerging, which through advertising, public relations, and the media promotes a kind of "medico-media hype." Even the most preliminary research findings are termed a breakthrough and spawn a press conference and a torrent of publicity.

And we are witnessing the medicalization of America: Uncle Sam has become Uncle Sam, M.D. Every infirmity and every ache seem to merit treatment. We have medicalized a whole range of human miseries and misfortunes that in the past were outside the doctor's jurisdiction, so that now almost anything that affects the workings of the body, or even the workings of the mind, may be given a medical diagnosis, including socially undesirable behavior such as drug abuse and poor school performance; unwanted physical characteristics such as baldness, infertility, and small breasts; and even the process of growing old itself. We can't accept the idea that some afflictions, as trivial as snoring and as terrible as brain cancer, remain incurable. And so more people go to doctors more often than they used to, and for milder conditions. It is not surprising then to discover that one-third of all the patients consulting doctors in general medical practice have no serious medical disorder. We are even patients when we know there is nothing at all wrong with us, since medicine now serves healthy people with health promotion and counseling, risk-factor assessment, and routine checkups.

At the same time, patienthood has become a more involved, more demanding, more difficult role. No longer does the patient leave things in the doctor's hands when he leaves the doctor's office. The patient is now an ancillary care-giver, a sort of student anatomist and apprentice physician who reads up on his disorder in the *Merck Manual* and manages his illness with do-it-yourself tests and self-administered treatments.

Doing Better

We are, in fact, an extraordinarily healthy society. America's current health status is unprecedented and is vastly superior to that of one hundred years ago. In 1888, food was scant for many, sanitation and living conditions were abysmal, water was often filthy. Work was exhausting. Life expectancy at birth was a little over forty. The great epidemics still cast a shadow across the country: yellow fever had struck only a few years before, and the specter of cholera was just lifting. And there was the usual toll taken by tuberculosis, typhoid, syphilis, smallpox, and diphtheria. Most medical treatment was performed by family members, neighbors, perhaps storekeepers. Even the wealthy only called a doctor for something that was very serious. Someone like Frank Carson would have faced a totally different world then.

Edward Thompson, for instance, awakes as usual on a wintry morning in 1888. He gets out of bed with considerable pain because, at forty-two, he has developed gout in his left foot. He does not plan to see a doctor about it, because in his opinion there is not much that can be done. And in any case, his gout, like his growing girth, indicates that he has achieved a level of prosperity to be proud of.

The house is cold and dark as Mr. Thompson makes his way to the dining room for a filling breakfast of cereal with sugar and heavy cream, brown-bread toast, doughnuts, boiled eggs, and coffee. The Irish maid coughs continually while serving and clearing the dishes. Her coughing has reminded him of the death of his young son from consumption a few years before, and he thinks of this as he walks down the snowy path to his carriage, which will take him to the bank where he works. He is very proud, however, of his three surviving children.

Two hours later, his wife Fanny fretfully rings for the maid to remove her untouched breakfast. At thirty-eight, she suffers from a prolapsed uterus after her seven pregnancies (three miscarriages), and dyspepsia. She has a series of errands to do this morning but really doesn't feel up to it. Besides, she is leery of the unhealthy cold air and the fetid odors of sewage in parts of her neighborhood. And everyone knows that germs—diphtheria, consumption, scarlet fever—travel by air.

Edward Thompson breaks up his workday with a leisurely lunch at his club. Savoring an aromatic Cuban cigar afterward, he reads the newspaper, noticing an article detailing the construction of a new, "modern" hospital No one would get him near such a place, God knows. Hospitals are places where immigrants and people with nowhere else to go, go to die. And doctors are hardly better. Quacks, many of them, he believes. Folding his paper, he walks heavily to the cloakroom, contemplating the remainder of his afternoon's work.

That evening, after a dinner of potato soup, boiled beef, boiled rice, canned vegetable salad, and bread pudding, he sits reading by the fire in the library. A glass of brandy is by his side to dull the knifelike pain in his gouty foot. He stares moodily into the fire and smiles slightly. He *does* have much to be thankful for. God grant him another generation to enjoy this good life.

The First Health Revolution

If Mr. Thompson had had to summon a doctor, he would have arrived with a stethoscope, a reflex hammer, a thermometer, and little else in his doctor's bag. The mainstays of medical treatment were bed rest, a nutritious diet, good nursing care, fresh air, and sunlight. Most of the pills, salves, and powders that he prescribed had no specific curative action. The doctor's armamentarium was limited to opium for pain and diarrhea, quinine for malaria, digitalis for heart failure, and cod liver oil for rickets. As Voltaire said, "The efficient physician is the man who successfully amuses his patient while nature effects a cure."

Only in the last fifty years or so has medicine acquired its astounding powers to diagnose and treat disease. Decades after Mr. Thompson's time, in 1928, we still had effective treatments or preventive measures for only 5 to 10 percent of the 360 most important medical diseases. By 1976 this figure had risen to between 50 and 55 percent.[1] A patient today has a far, far better chance of receiving an effective and specific treatment for his ailment than he did fifty years ago.

An earthshaking discovery made between 1890 and 1894 was one of the first milestones in this health revolution. French and German bacteriologists isolated the diphtheria bacterium, infected horses with it, and then collected the antibodies that the horses' immune systems manufactured to combat the infection. When these antibodies were then injected into humans, those people became immune to diphtheria. Man had unearthed a specific cause for a specific disease and had then devised an invincible means of protection against it. The floodgates were thrown open.

In 1936, the first of the sulfa drugs was found to cure streptococcal infections; never before had we been able to stop an infection outright, and now it could be done simply with the use of a few tablets.[2] The impact of this is hard to appreciate today. Before 1936, a simple splinter in one's finger could give way to a raging infection that would travel rapidly through the soft tissues of the fingers and hand. Red streaks might appear running up the arm, and distant lymph nodes could become inflamed and painful as the infection spread. If the patient was to survive at all, or even to retain the use of his fingers and hand, he had to go through months of hot soaks and applications of antiseptics. But the sulfa drugs ended this. Infected cuts simply dried up, and dreaded diseases such as meningitis could be stopped.

In the early 1940s, an even greater "wonder drug," penicillin, was discovered. Suddenly we could cure pneumonia, one of the great killers of young men and women, and rheumatic fever, which had previously left many with permanently damaged hearts. After penicillin came a deluge of different antibiotics, including, in 1944, streptomycin, which was effective against tuberculosis, the Western world's number-one killer.

In the 1950s and 1960s came other stunning advances. Cortisone and other hormones were synthesized and then administered to treat arthritis and inflammatory bowel disease. We developed drugs to lower blood pressure, to correct an irregular heart rhythm, to thin the blood, to halt Parkinson's disease, to prevent epileptic seizures, to control depression and schizophrenia. With the development of chemotherapy and radiation therapy, we have made strides against many cancers, including childhood leukemias and Hodgkin's disease.

Surgery has witnessed the same revolution. Modern surgery has only been in existence for the last 100 to 150 years, made possible by the discovery of general anesthesia in the first half of the nineteenth century, the development of techniques to combat surgical blood loss and shock, and the use of aseptic techniques to control germs and avoid postoperative infections. Surgeons could now enter the body cavities to remove gallstones and kidney stones, to sew up stomach ulcers, to remove tumors of the bowel and of the brain.[3] More recently, surgical techniques have been coupled with astounding new technologies: heart-lung machines, kidney-dialysis machines, ultrasound, pacemakers, and lasers. There has indeed been a profound revolution in biomedical science, with the creation of modern medical and surgical care as we know it.

The Second Health Revolution

Recently, we have had a second health revolution—a revolution in preventive medicine and health promotion. In 1979, the U.S. Surgeon General, Dr. Julius Richmond, issued a report entitled "Healthy People" in which it was estimated that one-half of current mortality was due to unhealthy behavior and lifestyles, and an additional 20 percent to environmental threats. The report placed the responsibility for health squarely on the individual, indicating that future improvements in health status would result more from altering unhealthy behavior patterns and lifestyles, curbing environmental hazards, and enhancing self-care than from personal medical care.

Evidence pointing toward this conclusion had been mounting. For example, studies of large populations disclosed that the number of healthy habits an individual practiced greatly affected life expectancy. In one study, people who practiced seven such habits were found to be healthier and live longer than those who practiced six, six more than five, and so on.[4] The life expectancy for a man who practiced zero to three of these habits was sixty-seven, while that for a man who practiced six to seven of them was seventy-eight, a whopping eleven years greater. Among women, the difference was seven years. The following "rules" for good health and longevity emerged: (1) eat three meals a day instead of snacking; (2) eat breakfast every day; (3) exercise moderately, for example, taking long walks, swimming, bicycling, and gardening three to five times a week; (4) sleep seven to eight hours a night; (5) do not smoke cigarettes; (6) drink alcohol in moderation; (7) maintain a moderate weight, neither drastically high nor low.

Other sorts of studies underscored the importance of lifestyle in general, lending support to the popular belief that how you live your life determines how long it will last. One study, for example, compared the inhabitants of Utah and Nevada.[5] These two states are contiguous, have similar climates and degrees of urbanization, and have residents with similar levels of income and education. But they have quite different lifestyles. Utah has many abstemious Mormons, whereas the lifestyle of many in Nevada centers upon the casino and entertainment areas of Reno and Las Vegas. The residents of Utah live significantly longer than their neighbors. For those between forty and forty-nine years old, for example, the death rate is 61 percent higher in Nevada than it is in Utah.

In recent decades, we have witnessed the collective health benefits of the behavioral changes that were made by large numbers of Americans. Our success in combating heart disease serves as an example. Between 1968 and 1976, the death rate from heart disease declined by 21 percent after years of increase, and that decline has continued. This dramatic success is broad-based: it is seen in men and women, in blacks and whites, and in all age groups. During this period we have developed new medical therapies for heart disease, such as coronary care units and cardiac surgery, and at the same time there has been widespread recognition of the importance of diet, fitness, and other aspects of one's lifestyle. Researchers have studied the beneficial contributions made by each type of advance—medical and behavioral—and have estimated that lifestyle changes accounted for more than one-half of the decline in deaths from heart disease.[6] When the dangers of saturated fats and elevated cholesterol became apparent, reduction in fat intake was advocated, and this resulted in declining cholesterol levels in the population as a whole. This reduction was estimated to account for 30 percent of the decline in deaths from heart attacks. Cigarette smoking was also identified as an important factor in mortality, and there was a significant decline in smoking between 1968 and 1976, especially among men. A quarter of the overall decline in deaths from heart disease is attributable to people having quit smoking. Finally, the importance of weight reduction and physical exercise in controlling heart disease was also discovered during this period, and there appears to have been a significant increase in the activity levels of the average American, which accounts for the remainder of the decline brought about by lifestyle changes.

Our National Health Status

The collective health of our nation is excellent, although it is true that there are sizable disadvantaged minorities whose health status remains shockingly poor. A child born in 1984 can expect to live to the age of 74.7. Life expectancy is greatest for white females (78.8 years) and least for non-white males (67.1). Between these extremes, nonwhite females live longer (75.3 years) than do white males (71 years).[7] Taking a historical view of life expectancy highlights our progress.[8] In 1900 the life expectancy at birth of the average American was 47.3. Over the next fifty years we made significant progress, but the gains in the last thirty-five years have been astonishing. Life expectancy in 1984 was a staggering 3.8 years greater than it was in 1970, only fourteen years before, and it was 6.5 years greater than it was in 1950.

Our increasing longevity is a manifestation of declining mortality. Death rates have declined by one-third during the last three decades, from 8.4 deaths per 1,000 people in 1950 to 5.5 deaths per 1,000 in 1984.[9] At our current age-specific death rates, seven out of ten people alive today will reach age 70, and four out of ten will celebrate their eightieth birthday. The mortality rates for ten of the fifteen most frequent causes of death have decreased, including heart disease, strokes, diabetes, and peptic ulcer. And while the age-adjusted death rates for some cancers have risen, we have accomplished a great deal and there is much to be proud of.

Infant mortality, another widely used measure of health status, has also been declining dramatically with each succeeding year.[10] From 1965 to 1982 we cut infant mortality rates in half! Since 1965, when the infant-mortality rate in the United States was 24.7 deaths per 1,000 live births, the rate has fallen quickly, by 4.4 percent a year on average. In 1982, infant mortality was down to 11.5 deaths per 1,000 live births, and by 1984 it had fallen to 10.6. The pace of the decline has slowed in recent years, however.[11] A large gap still persists in the rate at which white and nonwhite infants die, but the accomplishments of the last twenty years are very substantial nonetheless.

Most Things Are Better by Morning

As significant as these advances in medicine are, they should not obscure our recognition of our innate biological tendency toward healthiness. The human body is actually a remarkably rugged and hardy biological system, one that is extraordinarily resistant to disease and injury. The reality is that we are resilient and adaptive, able to maintain our physical integrity by healing our wounds and repairing internal damage. Three kinds of self-protective mechanisms make this so: the organism as a whole can take defensive action; each organ system has specific protective and healing mechanisms; and individual cells carry out their own reparative processes.

At the highest level, our ability to perceive the environment and respond to it keeps us healthy.[12] We can spot potential hazards and avoid them before they are upon us. For example, if food smells spoiled, we do not eat it and thereby avert food poisoning. Seeing a burner on the stove glowing red, we know that it is too hot to touch and avoid a burn. And although we think of pain as pathological and noxious, pain is actually an early-warning system that alerts us to injury or disease so that the body can mobilize its healing powers and marshal its resistance before further damage ensues. Physicians are all too familiar with the serious injuries that can occur when pain perception is impaired; for example, diabetics who have lost sensation in their legs often develop severe infections and extensive injuries because pain has not warned them that something is wrong.

Each organ system also has its own unique self-protective mechanisms. The immune system coordinates and directs the body's war against toxic substances and infectious agents by orchestrating the inflammatory response. Inflammation, which we tend to think of as pathological, is actually protective because it contains tissue damage and then promotes healing and rebuilding. Other organ systems have their own defenses: the respiratory tract responds to inhaled irritants, like smoke, by coughing, which expels the irritant; the stomach reacts to poisons by vomiting them up, in effect jettisoning them before they can do more harm; if a major blood vessel is cut, a clot forms at the site and the muscular wall of the artery automatically goes into spasm, both of which minimize blood loss.

And finally, healing occurs at the cellular level. Cells have their own built-in capacity to fight off disease and repair damage: they attack, engulf, and extrude foreign bodies and invading microorganisms. And they replace their own depleted ranks by dividing to create more cells just like those that have been killed. Many kinds of cells, such as bone, skin, and blood, regenerate themselves by cell division after tissue death or loss.

We live in a veritable sea of microorganisms, many eminently capable of making us sick. Yet for the most part, we never succumb to them. Pneumococcus, for example, the bacterium that causes pneumonia, can be found in the throats of most healthy people. It is our innate resistance to disease that prevents these bacteria from establishing themselves in our lungs and making us clinically sick. The noteworthy phenomenon is not that a few people come down with pneumonia, but that most of us do not. It is easy to lose sight of this basic fact—that health is the rule and sickness the exception, rather than vice versa. The real question is not what makes us occasionally fall ill, but rather what keeps us healthy so much of the time. As Lewis Thomas says in *The Lives of a Cell,* "The great secret . . . is that most things get better by themselves. Most things, in fact, are better by morning."[13]

Feeling Worse

But much like Frank Carson, many Americans have lost sight of this inherent healthiness. While we have been very successful in improving our health status as a society, a commensurate subjective feeling of healthiness has proven elusive. Indeed, the harder we try to hit the bull's eye, the more it seems that we are missing the mark. We seem unable to enjoy our good health, to translate it into feelings of well-being and physical security. Rather, there is a sense of "disease" in the air. We are disturbed by minor ailments, haunted by the possibility of sickness, and plagued by a seeming necessity for constant medical attention. In nationwide polls, Americans say they are less satisfied with their health and their physical condition than they were; they are now more disturbed and more disabled by minor ailments and report that their everyday illnesses seem to last longer than formerly.

We are pursuing perfect health and yet living all the while like invalids. We act as if perpetually poised on the brink of breakdown, while denying it at the same time. We don't live exuberantly but apprehensively, as if our bodies are dormant adversaries, programmed for betrayal at any moment. In spite of all the attention and care we lavish on the body, it still seems inherently vulnerable to disease and injury, fragile and in constant jeopardy.

We fear not just for our health, but for our physical safety in general, since disease is only one of the corporeal threats to which we feel so vulnerable. There are environmental carcinogens and pesticides in our food, occupational hazards in the workplace, and industrial wastes in our tap water. There are drunk drivers cruising the roads and the senseless mayhem of cyanide-laced painkillers on store shelves. And our homes are no safer, with radon gas accumulating in the basement, formaldehyde fumes leaking out from behind walls covered with lead paint, and asbestos fibers falling from the ceilings. Even the most benign consumer products are festooned with stickers warning of their lethal possibilities. Along with this growing feeling of being unsafe is a rising intolerance of all physical risk, no matter how small a threat it poses. In our absolute intolerance of medical uncertainty and our faultfinding reactions to some accidental injuries, we manifest not just the wish to minimize risk, but the belief that we can eliminate it entirely.

Prisoners of Health

This book is about the pursuit of health. How can a personal and societal crusade to conquer disease paradoxically leave us feeling dis-eased? How can we do a better job of translating our objective medical advances into greater subjective feelings of healthiness?

To unravel this paradox, we need first to explore the psychology of health, to understand how people experience their bodies and think about illness. The feeling of total healthiness requires more than objective physical health, for it depends upon your beliefs about your health, your emotional state of mind, and what your life circumstances are like at the time. Perceiving bodily symptoms and deciding that you are sick is actually a very tricky business. People can be healthy but feel ill, and they can be diseased and yet feel fine. Two different people with the same disease can have totally different levels of suffering and report totally different symptoms. It is because the perception of health is so subjective that its pursuit can imprison us.

Knowing about the personal psychology of health, we will then be in a position to examine our society's heightened health consciousness and its perplexing consequences. We will explore why Americans are so concerned with their health and medical care at this particular time in our history and suggest where it will lead.

CHAPTER 2

How We Perceive Symptoms

ON THE MORNING of May 21, 1979, two hundred and twenty-four elementary-school pupils assembled in their school auditorium in Norwood, Massachusetts.[1] They were watching a play by the sixth graders, when suddenly one of the performers became dizzy and fell from the stage, cutting his chin. Several of the students in the front row immediately felt dizzy, weak, faint, and developed shaking chills. Their "illness" rapidly spread to those near them. The afflicted children were placed on the auditorium floor and covered with blankets. As panic spread, the fire department was called. An environmental contaminant was suspected and the building evacuated. The illness continued to spread and soon the number of sick children exceeded the capacity of emergency vehicles to transport them to hospitals. A team of physicians and nurses was dispatched to the school. Thirty-four children were taken to the hospital and more than forty were treated at the scene. But examining physicians could find nothing wrong with any of the children, other than mild signs of anxiety. Within four hours the epidemic was over. No disease agent, such as a virus or bacterium, was ever discovered, even though the school's water, milk, cafeteria, and ventilation system were all carefully tested.

This is an example of what is called mass or epidemic hysteria. Physical symptoms suddenly spread through a group of people, rapidly making them all sick, but the symptoms are not caused by a real disease. They are psychological in origin. They tend to be vague or generalized, such as nausea, dizziness, hot or cold flashes, or feeling faint. Outbreaks occur among people who are in close proximity, such as pupils at a boarding school, campers at a summer camp, or participants in a weekend retreat. The symptoms are first manifested by someone who is particularly prominent in the group and then spread to others nearby, as if contagion could occur through sight and sound.

The explanation of epidemic hysteria lies in the powerful influence that situation and circumstance have on our perception of bodily sensations. If someone beside you suddenly feels dizzy and weak, you check yourself for these same symptoms. Mild, ambiguous sensations such as lightheadedness, a rapid heartbeat, or feeling chilled, which you would otherwise have ignored, suddenly seem ominous, since they are now interpreted as signs of a contagious disease overwhelming everyone around you. Now you think you are falling ill, and your anxiety produces its own set of physical symptoms that are then mistaken for additional evidence that you are sick. You feel worse and worse.

In this chapter we will consider how we perceive and experience symptoms—what makes them feel better and what makes them feel worse. When you notice a pain in your back, or a stuffy nose, what determines how uncomfortable you are? How do you decide which bodily sensations are worthy of your attention or concern? In succeeding chapters we will go on to examine *who* feels their symptoms most intensely, and then *why* people experience physical suffering when there is no physical cause.

Four factors can make you amplify bodily symptoms: the circumstances you are in at the time; your beliefs about what is causing them; how much attention you pay to them; and your mood. To appreciate how these four factors operate in our daily lives, we must first appreciate how much trivial illness we experience every day.

Everyday Illness

When people become alarmed about their health, they already have at hand a panoply of mild bodily sensations to focus upon. Lots of insignificant, benign illness comes and goes from day to day: a sore inside the cheek, a rash, poor appetite, diarrhea. Thus as we become more health conscious we need only to focus on this welter of mild symptoms and trivial illnesses to substantiate our apprehension. Everyday illness, in other words, is the fertile soil onto which health concerns fall and take root.

If we ask healthy people to keep a careful diary of all the symptoms they experience, they record stuffy and runny noses, coughing, fatigue, headaches, corns and calluses, rashes, palpitations, and myriad other complaints. The typical adult in such a study records a symptom of illness on one day out of every four and has about eighty symptomatic episodes per year.[2] Only about 15 percent of people are without any symptoms over a period of fourteen days.[3] If we examine this phenomenon of everyday illness more comprehensively by judging the overall health status of a typical sample of adults, we find that 28 percent have one or more chronic medical disorders, another 28 percent have at least one symptomatic complaint, and 15 percent consider themselves to be significantly disabled.[4] The reality, then, is that most of the time, most of us are neither gravely ill nor totally symptom-free. Rather, we live midway between these extremes, experiencing the constant wear and tear of mild, nagging infirmities and transient, self-limited disorders.[5]

We can think of these benign symptoms and trivial illnesses as a kind of background noise that we usually ignore. At certain times we become more sensitive to, and more aware of, this background noise, and it becomes bothersome. At these times, we focus on these mild sensations and amplify them into intense, alarming symptoms that make us think we're really sick.

We can now discuss in turn the four factors that cause us

to amplify the background noise of everyday illness: circumstances, beliefs, attention, and mood.

Circumstances

If someone in your family has a cold, the next time you sneeze you will notice it and are likely to conclude that you have caught the cold too. But if no one around you were ill, you would hardly notice having sneezed. How a person experiences a sensation, and even whether he perceives it at all, depends upon the circumstances he is in at the time. If you are waiting in your office for someone who is late, you will hear footsteps in the hallway that you would not have noticed otherwise. Situation and setting are most influential when the bodily symptom is vague and ambiguous (such as loss of appetite, fatigue, or insomnia), and when there is no obvious cause to explain it (as there is when you injure yourself, for example).

The phenomenon known as battlefield anesthesia dramatically illustrates the importance of circumstances. Soldiers in the heat of battle can disregard, and even be utterly oblivious to, severe wounds. It is not until the battle is over that the individual perceives his injury. In a classic investigation of this, the pain experiences of soldiers wounded in the World War II battle at Anzio Beachhead were compared with those of civilians with similar wounds that resulted from surgery.[6] The soldiers reported much less pain than their civilian counterparts, and they used fewer painkillers. Indeed, though the soldiers had extensive wounds, less than one-quarter said they had enough pain to want anything done about it.

The differing perceptions of similar symptoms are attributable to the differing contexts. A nonfatal wound sustained in military combat is an anticipated, perhaps even welcome, event. There may be a certain amount of glory associated with it; it also means that the soldier has escaped with his life from mortal combat; and it provides a legitimate ticket away from the front lines. For the civilian, on the other hand, accidental trauma is unexpected, calamitous, and totally unlike anything happening to others around him. If occasioned by surgery, as in this case, there is also the frightening specter of the disease being treated. From this study it was concluded, "Something other than extent or degree of wounding is of principal importance in the pain experienced. . . . The intensity of suffering is largely determined by what the pain means to the patient."[7]

Circumstances cause us to amplify or reduce bodily symptoms in more pedestrian situations as well. For example, a backache seems worse when you are facing an onerous day of household chores than it does when you are about to go fishing with friends. Banging your shin while groping your way to the bathroom in the middle of the night is more painful than the same bruise sustained while having a great time skiing. Children manifest the same phenomenon: their headaches and stomach aches invariably intensify when they are asked to do something they prefer to avoid, such as clearing the dishes or finishing their homework. How often we have been shown a minuscule, or even invisible, "cut" on a tiny finger just at the moment we are leaving our young children with a baby-sitter.

A number of psychology experiments have been devised to study the way context influences our experience of somatic (bodily) symptoms. They show that what we *expect* to be feeling powerfully shapes what we *do* feel. One such study examined people's perceptions of their skin temperature, while actually recording it at the same time.[8] The subjects were given earphones and told they would be hearing "ultrasonic noise." Some subjects were told that this would raise skin temperature slightly while others were told that it would lower it. Though no changes in skin temperature actually occurred, subjects felt that their skin temperatures had moved up or down according to what they had been told to expect.

Circumstances and setting also lead people to ignore certain perceptions and to decide that they are not the symptoms of disease. If a somatic sensation is common among the people around you, then you are unlikely to conclude that it is symptomatic of a disease when you experience it. Backaches, for example, are not considered abnormal or a symptom of disease by laborers whose work involves much heavy lifting. Similarly, diarrhea is not noteworthy among poor people whose inadequate nutrition and sanitation cause widespread gastrointestinal disorder.

Beliefs

The thoughts or beliefs that a person has about a physical symptom can make it feel worse. Our first thoughts, once we become aware of a symptom, usually center on imagining its cause. You may suspect a benign cause such as overwork, physical exertion, insufficient sleep, aging, or a dietary indiscretion. Or you may attribute your symptom to a disease, one that may or may not have been diagnosed already. Your suspicion that a bodily sensation is caused by a serious disease amplifies the sensation: a stomach ache feels worse if you fear it is caused by stomach cancer than if you think it results from a meal that was too spicy. So in a sense, believing a symptom is serious can cause it to be so.

Beyond affecting how intense our symptoms seem, our beliefs about a symptom also affect which sensations we will notice subsequently and how we will interpret them. Once you have determined a cause for a sensation, then you will selectively screen future sensations for information to confirm your theory, and you may disregard information that doesn't fit it. If you are walking along a trail in the woods and glimpse a long, thin, dark form at the edge of the trail, you might conclude that it is a dead branch or a snake. If you think it is a snake, then you will interpret a rustling sound as the snake moving, providing further confirmation of your hypothesis. On the other hand, if you think you saw a branch, then you might attribute the rustling sound to a breeze in the trees and glance up to see whether the leaves are fluttering. With a bodily sensation, the process is the same: once someone has commented that you look pale, you take normal breathlessness after climbing stairs as evidence that you are ill.

Thus cognitive schemes are self-perpetuating. Once you believe you have a serious disease, then all future sensations are interpreted to confirm it. Once formed, in other words, the attribution, whether correct or not, tends to persist, because subsequent normal bodily sensations are taken as further evidence of disease. This is what happened to Frank Carson. After he began to suspect he had a brain tumor, his headaches seemed worse. Unrelated symptoms, such as blurry vision when he was tired, took on an ominous new meaning because he imagined that they were symptoms of a spreading tumor.

In a study among patients who had had a chest X ray and were informed that further investigation was necessary because of a possible abnormality, one-tenth developed new or increased symptoms that they thought were caused by heart disease.[9] If you think an X ray has revealed some problem with your heart, then normal sensations in your chest that you might otherwise have ignored take on an entirely different meaning and consequently become more severe.

Experiments have shown that pain can be ameliorated when people believe that ancillary symptoms are caused by a pill just taken rather than being related to the pain.[10] Researchers gave placebos (inactive pills) to subjects who had volunteered to receive painful electric shocks. Some subjects were told that the pill would cause a pounding heart, a faster respiratory rate, and butterflies in the stomach—symptoms that do in fact accompany pain. Others were told that the placebo would cause a different set of symptoms, ones that do not accompany the pain of the electric shock. The subjects who believed that all their bodily symptoms were caused by the pill they had taken found the shocks less painful and tolerated more of them than the people who thought that all their symptoms were caused by the shocks themselves.

Similar work has been done with insomniacs who complain of an anxious alertness and a nervous arousal when they are trying unsuccessfully to fall asleep. They notice an increased heart rate, a sense of physical tension, racing thoughts, "knots" in the stomach, and other unpleasant sensations. These symptoms make them feel as if their minds are getting the best of them. When given a pill that they believe causes these symptoms, insomniacs are able to fall asleep.[11] This is because the symptoms of insomnia seem less disturbing if they believe they're caused by a neutral external agent (the pill) rather than by their own sleep problem. Sleeplessness can become a vicious cycle: anxiety and frustration about falling asleep increase the insomniac's alertness and arousal, which then makes it even harder for him to fall asleep. This leads to further upset, and the cycle continues. But as the experiment shows, if the insomniac believes that the disturbing symptoms he feels are not his fault but rather are due to the pill he has taken, he becomes less upset with himself for the difficulty he is having in falling asleep. This lowering of arousal allows him to doze off.

Confusion and ignorance about which bodily symptoms are caused by disease and which are not is very important in clinical medicine. The recuperation of heart-attack victims is often hindered by their mistaken belief that benign symptoms such as breathlessness when exercising, and weakness (which is normal after prolonged bed rest) are evidence of continuing active heart disease. This impedes the resumption of an active and full life and promotes invalidism, as can be seen in the following story.

Ruth Bear, a fifty-four-year-old single woman who worked stocking shelves in a clothing store, was discharged after a ten-day hospitalization for an uncomplicated heart attack.

Her physician saw no obstacles to a gradual resumption of full activity. However, at the time of her first follow-up visit, she seemed demoralized, was not tending her vegetable garden, and talked of giving up her job, which she had always enjoyed immensely and taken great pride in. Her doctor noticed that she still had on the plastic identification bracelet she had worn in the hospital. When he mentioned it, she explained, "They forgot to cut it off me when I was discharged and I didn't get around to cutting it off. . . . Maybe I'll flop over again and with this bracelet they'll know to bring me right here."

Miss Bear went on to reveal that she was frightened by symptoms she had experienced since her discharge from the hospital: she was weak and breathless after walking to the corner to buy a newspaper and noticed palpitations when she got up at night to go to the bathroom. Though these are common complaints during the recovery from any major illness, Ruth thought they indicated that her heart disease was progressing. She therefore thought that a second heart attack was imminent and feared that every step she took might be her last. A careful discussion of this misunderstanding of her symptoms was followed by an uneventful recovery. This woman's reactions illustrate how a patient's beliefs about her symptoms can make the difference between discomfort and comfort, between recuperation and invalidism.

Attention

Paying attention to a symptom amplifies it, while distractions reduce it. Whenever Frank Carson got a headache he would focus on it, checking to see if the pain traveled in any direction, comparing it with the previous one, and so on. And the more he paid attention to it, the more meticulously and continuously he observed it, the more intense and unpleasant it grew. This effect of attention upon sensation can readily be observed. Take a moment to concentrate upon the temperature of your hands. Try to imagine that the right is getting warmer and the left is getting colder. If you really concentrate on this sensation, after a few seconds you will actually begin to feel that your right hand is warming up and your left is cooling off. To take another illustration of the power of attention, if you are totally engrossed in a movie, you can become oblivious to the pain of your recently sprained ankle. It is only when the theater lights come up and you are jolted out of your reverie that the pain returns.

Psychology experiments have confirmed that concentrating upon one's body increases the number of symptoms that will be reported, and that concentrating on a particular bodily sensation intensifies it.[12] Interestingly, other research has shown that paying increased attention to one's *performance* on a variety of tasks leads to a lower opinion of one's ability.[13] Thus it may be an inherent tendency of the human mind that the more you reflect upon your characteristics, the more negatively you assess them. Self-scrutiny apparently leads to self-criticism.

Coughing, yawning, itching, and pain are symptoms that are particularly sensitive to attention. Almost everyone has observed how yawning seems to be contagious. And next time you are with others in a social situation, scratch yourself and watch to see how many other people scratch themselves soon after. You have given a subliminal suggestion that normal bodily sensations seem uncomfortable and itchy. The same thing goes for coughing. When someone near you coughs, it calls your attention to your own throat; soon you begin to feel a tickling or dry sensation, an itchiness or scratchiness, and before you know it, you find yourself clearing your throat and then coughing. You can get the same effect just by thinking about your throat for a moment as you read this. Performers know that coughing at plays and concerts occurs in discrete epidemics. Someone begins, possibly because of illness, and then rapidly "recruits" those sitting nearby. After the outbreak dies down, another one will begin elsewhere in the audience. The infectious agent in this epidemic is attention.

This phenomenon has been studied. An audience rated successive thirty-second segments of a movie for their interest.[14] The film was then shown to another audience and the number of coughs in each half-minute segment were counted. There was a clear inverse relationship: the less interesting the film, the more coughing occurred. Boring parts of the film offered less external distraction and at these times people were more likely to notice their internal bodily sensations.

A common experiment to test pain tolerance is the cold pressor test. Here the subject immerses his hand in a bucket of ice-cold water. Individuals tolerate the cold water longer if they are looking at distracting scenes than if they are looking at their own hands in the water. Studies of people having dental extractions revealed the same thing. After several teeth were pulled, the patients were periodically asked to report how much pain they were experiencing. At the end of two hours, those who rated their pain experience every twenty minutes reported more intense pain than those who had rated their pain only once before.[15]

Physicians see this phenomenon in hospitalized patients who are in pain, for example, patients who are recuperating from surgery. They complain more, and request more analgesic medicine, at night when there is less external stimulation to distract them. During the day there are visitors to see, hospital staff to chat with, and activities such as meals or physical therapy or going to other hospital floors for tests. These sensory inputs capture the patients' attention, and bodily symptoms diminish.

Many joggers, particularly beginners rather than marathoners, find that concentrating on subjects or events unrelated to running increases their exertional tolerance. In one experiment, subjects exercised on a treadmill; some listened through earphones to interesting bits of conversation, while others listened to the sound of their own labored breathing.[16] After exercising, the groups of subjects did not differ in objective measures such as heart rate or blood pressure, but they did differ significantly in their subjective reports of physical symptoms such as fatigue, racing heart, and sweating. Those who heard their own breathing reported being most bothered by these physical symptoms. A similar phenomenon seems to occur among assembly-line workers: those with the most boring, repetitive, and undemanding jobs report more physical symptoms, take more aspirin, and have more medical absences.

Hypnosis is a form of intense concentration in which there is a dramatic decrease in the awareness of external stimuli. It can produce profound anesthesia to pain and other bodily discomfort. Highly hypnotizable people can even undergo major surgery without any anesthesia other than deep hypnosis. Under hypnosis the subject focuses his attention on some pleasurable mental image, making the pain less noxious because he disregards it. The sensation of pain remains, but the associated suffering and discomfort are reduced so that the pain feels more like a tingling or numbness. Other trance states, such as the trance dancing seen in some nonindustrialized cultures, have the same effect. Trance dancers may walk on hot coals, for instance, without feeling any pain. While this is a novel example, the general phenomenon is common in everyday life: paying attention to discomfort worsens it and distraction ameliorates it.

Moods

Certain moods cause us to amplify our symptoms. Frank Carson was frightened, and when filtered through this veil of apprehension, a feeling of mild pressure became a throbbing, boring ache, and lightheadedness seemed like a loss of consciousness.

There is a general relationship between physical distress and psychological distress. To put it simply, if you experience a lot of mental discomfort, you are likely to experience a lot of physical discomfort too. People who report many bodily symptoms report many psychological symptoms as well, such as feeling more moody, more high-strung, and more easily hurt.[17] Several mechanisms account for this. First of all, strong emotions produce physiological changes throughout the body: perspiration, a pounding and racing heart, frequent urination, diarrhea, to name a few. Sadness, for example, produces a "choked-up" sensation in the throat and "heartache"; fear brings on a pounding heart and a sudden weakness in the legs; rage makes people's faces feel hot and their muscles tense. And second, some unpleasant moods, such as anxiety and depression, cause people to amplify any preexisting bodily symptoms they may have. Thus when people are emotionally upset, their physical symptoms become more severe.

The more anxious a person is, the more sensitive he is to a mildly painful stimulus such as a pinprick, and the lower is his tolerance of severe pain. A sore throat, for example, can become excruciating when you are very anxious about speaking in public. The sensitivity to all bodily sensations is heightened in this state because anxious people are self-conscious, aroused, and keyed up, and thus more attentive to what is going on in their bodies. In addition to their heightened somatic sensitivity, people who are chronically anxious or tense for long periods develop several characteristic symptoms, such as abdominal cramps, sore muscles, and profuse sweating.

The following clinical case illustrates how anxiety amplifies symptoms. Bill Strasser had an acute anxiety attack while hospitalized for surgery on his badly fractured leg. His panic occurred when an alarm rang on a monitor connected to the patient in the bed beside him (it turned out to be a false alarm). Bill had been in the submarine service during the Korean War, serving as a damage-control officer. His job, should his submarine be hit, was to close watertight bulkheads that sealed off the damaged compartment and prevented flooding of the entire vessel. The final step in this procedure was to sound an alarm to warn anyone still in the damaged area that it was about to be sealed off from the rest of the ship. In his delirious state in the hospital, Bill confused the alarm in the intensive-care unit with the alarm used on the submarine, and he panicked, terrified that he was about to be sealed off behind a bulkhead in a compartment flooding with seawater. He tried to climb out of bed to escape, but his plaster cast immobilized him. In trying to get out of bed he spilled the water from his pitcher on himself and mistook this for the ocean pouring into the submarine, heightening his terror.

After his discharge from the hospital, Bill had to remain immobilized in bed at home while his leg healed. Over the succeeding weeks, he experienced more acute anxiety attacks. He was terrified at being alone in his house and unable to escape should a disaster occur. Moreover, his anxiety was causing him to amplify mild symptoms and complaints. A normal twinge in the muscles of his chest seemed to him like the crushing chest pain of a heart attack, and he kept feeling as if he were choking and unable to take in a deep enough breath. He began to monitor himself closely for any signs of an impending heart attack or blood clot in his lungs. Though his heart and lungs were in fact perfectly normal, he counted his respiratory rate, took his pulse and blood pressure, and recorded them religiously. Only as he became able to get up and around did his anxiety decline, and along with it his somatic complaints.

Depression also causes people to worry about their health and to amplify their bodily sensations. But rather than turning inward in apprehension and alarm, the depressed individual's self-scrutiny has a dejected, pessimistic, and despondent quality. He believes that he deserves to be sick, is not worth treating, and has little hope of recovery. Expecting the worst, the depressed person thinks that a bout of constipation must indicate a tumor of the colon.

While schizophrenia is not a mood per se, it does illustrate how profoundly emotional distress affects our perception of our bodies. Schizophrenia is a serious disorder in which thinking is disorganized and many emotions are inappropriate. Hallucinations and delusions (false, fixed beliefs) are usually present. Schizophrenics are also remarkably insensitive to physical discomfort. They can remain immobile for hours, locked in rigid and contorted body postures. Loud noises seem to go unnoticed. Severe pain (such as that of acute appendicitis) is easily tolerated, and schizophrenics sometimes mutilate themselves without seeming to feel it. Pain-sensitivity tests confirm these observations. The mechanism behind this phenomenon is not known, but it illustrates how powerfully psychological states can alter the perception of bodily symptoms.

Amplifiers Can Make Things Worse

Much of the time we are experiencing one insignificant bodily symptom or another. We amplify some of these mild sensations and reduce others. We've discussed the factors that help determine how bad a given symptom feels: the circumstances we are in, the beliefs and information (or misinformation) we have about the sensation, how much attention we give it, and what our mood is at the time that we experience it.

Circumstances, beliefs, attention, and mood can themselves all be influenced by the people around us, by our social environment. These amplifiers thus function as mediators through which cultural attitudes, values, and beliefs shape our own personal experience of illness and our perception of our bodies. These four factors, and their sensitivity to cultural influences, help explain how the pursuit of health can become paradoxical. A health-conscious culture focuses our attention on our bodies, engenders a mood of alarm about health matters, creates an atmosphere of disease omnipresence, and furnishes the suggestion that minor symptoms are caused by serious diseases. In so doing, our culture teaches each of us to notice more bodily symptoms and to feel more ill. Thus, beyond a certain point, a heightened health consciousness may engender more bodily discomfort and unease by supplying a context, a belief system, an attentional focus, and an apprehensive mood, which all magnify health concerns and bodily symptoms.

CHAPTER 3

Who Feels Healthy and Who Feels Sick

WHEN IT COMES TO FEELING ILL, your mind is not above playing tricks on you. As John Milton wrote in *Paradise Lost,* "The mind is its own place and in itself can make a Heaven of Hell, a Hell of Heaven." Our subjective feelings of healthiness do not correspond very closely to how healthy we actually are because we are inaccurate reporters of what is going on inside our bodies.

Thus there is an important distinction between the biological state of health and the mental perception of healthiness. The terms *disease* and *illness* make this distinction. *Disease* refers to a physical or chemical abnormality; it is a biological process. Illness, on the other hand, is your conscious experience of disease. *Illness* refers to the suffering and disability you experience, to the personal meaning and significance the disease has for you. In short, illness is what you feel, while disease is what you have. Two different people with the same disease may experience two entirely different sets of symptoms—different illnesses. And while one person may be in agony with a bee sting, another bears terminal bone cancer with quiet and calm stoicism.

Who tends to feel sicker and suffer more, and who feels healthier and has fewer symptoms? Before answering this question, we must first look at the way the nervous system processes bodily sensations.

The Subjectivity of Symptoms

Incoming sensations from all over the body are conducted by nerves to the spinal cord and then up to the brain. Thus the brain is continually bombarded with sensory information about normal bodily processes, such as digestion or breathing, and about minor problems, such as a cramp, an itch, or a stiff joint. Superimposed upon this continuous "background noise" are the occasional signals of a serious disease or injury.

The brain actively sifts, colors, and filters all the signals it receives, amplifying some, damping down others. Many sensations never ascend to a high enough level in the brain to reach conscious awareness. Thus we may be totally unaware of our heart beating or of our stomach contracting, we may not notice a minor cut until we accidentally see the blood, or we may scratch an itch without even realizing it. But some sensations are forwarded to higher levels in the brain. Here they are combined with other sensory input, integrated with memories of past experience, evaluated in light of relevant knowledge, and embellished with emotion. Thus invested with meaning and feeling, the original perception is transformed into a complete conscious experience.

In a similar way, the brain transforms and interprets sights, sounds, and smells. In viewing Picasso's *Guernica,* we "see" more than a collection of different pigments in different positions on a canvas, more than shapes and colors. In seeing the painting, we experience pain, horror, and sorrow. Upon the visual image that enters the brain from the canvas, we superimpose our personal experiences of terror, our memories, and other images of war we have seen. Similarly, a Beethoven symphony is more than sound waves. It is an experience of poetry and of awe, of mood and of memory, which is created in the listener's brain. So the process of perception, whether it be of the body or of a work of art, is variable and subjective. Sensation is transmuted into experience.

When Things Are Not What They Seem

Different people with the same medical disorder may have very different symptoms. Peptic ulcer is a good example. In one study, patients were treated with large doses of antacids, and the size of the ulcers in their stomachs was determined by X ray before and after treatment.[1] The antacids proved effective in healing the ulcers, but what is most striking from our point of view was the lack of a relationship between ulcer healing and symptom relief. Forty-eight percent of the patients who still complained of their symptoms were found to be ulcer-free after treatment. Conversely, 33 percent of the patients who reported their symptoms gone still showed active ulcers when X-rayed. In other words, patients whose ulcers had healed were no more likely to become symptom-free than patients whose ulcers did not heal. Studies of the pain resulting from arthritis of the spine, and of patients with asthma and diabetes, also show that the extent of a patient's disease is a poor predictor of how much distress the patient reports.

The placebo effect illustrates this discrepancy between the objective disease and the subjective illness. Medications often produce symptom relief even when they do not have a specific chemical action against the particular disease that is being treated. This is called the placebo effect. A placebo is a pill that is given with the intention of treating a medical disease, but which has no specific biological or chemical activity against the condition. A sugar pill is an example of a placebo, but medical procedures and even surgical operations can be placebos as well, as long as they have no specific curative action. The placebo effect has been the doctor's major therapeutic tool through most of history. Until the mid-1800s, very few of his remedies had any specific curative action. And yet there is ample evidence that many people treated with these placebo remedies did improve.

The patient believes that the placebo is effective and therefore expects relief. And, despite the fact that it is inert, the placebo does indeed relieve the symptoms of a wide range of medical disorders. About 35 percent of people will obtain symptomatic relief with a placebo. Placebos are effective in treating postoperative pain, chest pain from heart disease, coughing, ulcer pain, migraine, and seasickness.

Even more remarkable, in considering the inexact correspondence between symptoms and disease, is the fact that 10 percent of patients receiving placebos report unpleasant side effects, such as dermatitis, diarrhea, and vomiting, just like those we find among people taking a chemically active drug. Some people even become addicted to placebos and have withdrawal symptoms when they suddenly stop taking them. And all this from simply ingesting a sugar pill.

The Range of Sensitivity to Disease

People fall along a spectrum in their sensitivity to bodily symptoms. Some people's somatic sensory experience is more intense, more intrusive, and more disturbing. They have a lower threshold for pain, and a lower tolerance of it, than other people do. Their brains amplify sensations that others would be unaware of, and they are made uncomfortable by sensations others find neutral. This may be a characteristic of their nervous systems, "hard-wired" into their brains from birth. We refer to these sensitive people as amplifiers, in contrast to reducers, who minimize and attenuate their bodily symptoms. Reducers are slow to perceive symptoms consciously, and they tend to respond by denying or ignoring them, unless of course they are quite severe. Bodily symptoms in general do not worry or alarm them.

Think what life is like for the amplifier. His nervous system augments normal bodily sensations and the trivial symptoms of minor illnesses. What some experience as a neutral feeling of pressure or tightness, the amplifier experiences as crushing pain. What to others is just being "out of breath" is to the amplifier an overwhelming sensation of smothering or choking. Where one woman feels an irregularity in the consistency of her breast tissue, the amplifier feels a larger "lump." The amplifier is like the princess in "The Princess and the Pea," who could not fall asleep atop even twenty mattresses because she was bothered by a pea beneath the bottom mattress.

People who amplify bodily sensation also appear to amplify other sensory modalities as well. Research suggests that people who amplify pain are also likely to amplify light and sound and touch. This tendency can be assessed in a number of ways. We can test a person's ability to perceive rapid flashes of light or faint sounds, for instance, or his ability to detect very mild pain that is produced experimentally.

In one particular experiment, amplification was studied by asking people to estimate the size and weight of objects placed in their hands while blindfolded.[2] Amplifiers who overestimated size and weight, when compared to people who underestimated them, were more sensitive to pain. When obstetricians rated the pain experiences of women giving birth, the women whom they judged to be having the most painful labors were the ones who tended to overestimate size and weight.

A provocative suggestion about reducers arose from this work. The most extreme reducers seem to be starved for sensory input and find this absence of stimulation very disturbing and unpleasant. Sensory deprivation and situations of monotony and confinement are agonizing for them. Among incarcerated prisoners, there is a subgroup who deliberately hurt or mutilate themselves when placed in solitary confinement. When tested, these prisoners were found to be extreme reducers. It may be that they are deliberately inducing pain as an antidote to the (for them) unbearable absence of sensation.

Do amplifiers and reducers differ in ways other than their perceptual sensitivity? We don't know much more about amplifiers and reducers, but we do know something about healthy people who report a greater number of disturbing bodily symptoms than others do. If we sample a large group of people, we find that some report many more symptoms than others. They also rate each of these symptoms as more severe than do people who report fewer symptoms. Seven characteristics determine whether you feel more symptomatic than the average person: age, gender, social class, ethnicity, marital status, degree of self-consciousness, and extent of feeling in control of your life.[3]

First of all, the older you are, in general, the more symptoms you report. And women consistently report more bodily symptoms and more minor illnesses than men. There are many psychological studies that, taken together, indicate that women are more sensitive to changes in their bodies, feel less healthy, take more medications, and think of themselves as more prone to illness than men. Several different explanations for this are possible. It may be, as we are arguing here, that women are just more innately sensitive to their bodily sensations than men—that they have the same amount of disease but find its symptoms more intense and more disturbing. Alternatively, their reports of more symptoms may reflect actual differences in the prevalence of minor disorders in men and women. Finally, it could be that women are simply more willing to acknowledge their symptoms and report them to someone else, to admit publicly to frailties and ailments.

Social class is another factor that differentiates people who are more and less symptomatic. Not surprisingly, the prevalence of medical symptoms and feelings of ill-health increase as social class declines. People who are more educated consider themselves to be in better health, and those with higher incomes are likewise inclined. This may be because the more affluent can afford more medical care and are thus objectively in better health.

Cultural and ethnic background can also affect who is more symptomatic and who less. It has been found that Jews and Italian-Americans exhibit an emotional and expressive response to pain, WASPs are more stoical, and Irish-Americans tend to deny pain outright.[4] When we compare the complaints of Italian and Irish patients with the same medical condition, the Irish report less pain, have symptoms that are more localized, and tend to understate their difficulties, while the Italians experience more dysfunction and more symptoms in more different bodily locations.[5] One study of chronic pain showed that Jews differed from Italians in that they were more concerned with the meaning of the pain experience and its prognostic implications, while the Italians were more concerned with obtaining relief for their discomfort.[6] The relative stoicism of WASP men has been attributed to an upbringing that stresses teaching young boys to take pain "like a man" and not to cry about it or to act like a "sissy."[7]

Finally, single people (over the age of thirty) are more symptomatic than their married counterparts.[8] This is in accord with a generalization that emerges from many survey studies in many different settings—that being married and being part of a tight and supportive social system make people feel more content, satisfied, and generally happier.

The tendency to report many bodily symptoms is also related to several personality characteristics, one of which is introspection. People who are highly introspective, self-aware, and self-conscious tend to appraise their health as worse than it is and to interpret stressful experiences and benign symptoms as evidence of disease.[9] (Such people also report more disturbing psychological symptoms as well.) Thus, after the Three Mile Island nuclear accident, highly introspective area residents interpreted the incident as more threatening and more serious and reported more physical and behavioral symptoms as a result than people who were less self-aware.[10]

Being more aware of oneself and of one's thoughts and moods has been termed private self-consciousness. But in addition, the tendency to be highly symptomatic has been associated with concern about how one presents oneself in public and with what other people think of one, a trait called public self-consciousness.[11] High symptom reporters feel, for example, that being physically attractive is extremely important. Thus the concern about the appearance of one's face and body, an emphasis upon how one looks, is related to concerns about health and physical symptoms of illness.

High symptom reporters also feel less able to control what happens to them in life and feel dependent upon other people or outside forces such as chance, luck, or fate.[12] They don't feel that their behavior will bring about the results they seek. In contrast, the more self-reliant people feel, the more they believe that they control their environment and their future and their health, the fewer bodily symptoms they are likely to report. Pain tends to feel milder to people who believe they have some control over its cause and who believe in general that they have the power to determine their life circumstances. This is part of the rationale behind the pain-control techniques used in natural childbirth, where the objective is to give the mother-to-be a sense of power and control over the pain experience.*

The feeling of personal control over our fate turns out to be an important component of psychological as well as physical well-being.[14] A sense of helplessness and ineffectiveness, of being a pawn, is not just physically disturbing; it is anxiety-provoking and depressing as well. People who feel in control are more satisfied with life and feel more positive emotionally.

---

* It is interesting to note that the sense of being in control may even affect actual health status, as well as feelings of physical well-being and symptom reports. In one study, for example, giving the elderly residents of a nursing home more of a say in their day-to-day lives (by allowing them to determine what they ate for meals, when phone calls would be forwarded to their rooms, and arranging their own furniture) dramatically lowered their mortality rate.[13]

Stoics and People Who Feel Healthy

We now move from considering the perception and reporting of bodily symptoms to a more general consideration of how people think about health and disease. Just as people are distributed along a spectrum of political interest ranging from the apathetic nonvoter to the political zealot, and just as there is a continuum of religious concern from the agnostic to the fanatical fundamentalist, so are people distributed along a smooth continuum of concern with health and illness. At one end is the stoic, at the other lies the hypochondriac.

Stoics don't pay much attention to their health status and they don't worry about getting sick. They may take their health for granted or regard it fatalistically, but either way, it is not a subject of great interest to them. When they actually are sick, they try to deny it to themselves and to those around them, minimizing the significance of any discomfort or disability. They hate being ill and don't tell people how bad they feel since they don't like to think of themselves as complainers and hate having others dote on them. Some people, for example, will continue to go about their business even after developing the crushing chest pain and sudden weakness that signal a heart attack to everyone else. They deny their condition and may delay visiting a physician until someone else—perhaps a spouse or a coworker—sweeps them up and literally transports them to an emergency room. Even then, with cold and clammy skin, an ashen face, and a weak pulse, the stoic may continue to deny he is in any distress or that anything is wrong.

At certain times in life, those of us who are not normally stoical experience a sort of temporary stoicism that allows us to glimpse what life is like for those who are. For example, sometimes we can temporarily repress a symptom of a serious disease. Jeanne Warren is an office worker who developed pain in her left shoulder. At first it only bothered her when she went swimming, which she had been doing regularly, so she stopped for a while and began jogging instead. She denied the pain, didn't tell anyone about it, and didn't even consider the possibility that it might be something serious. Though she kept moving her arm as much as she could, eventually she could barely put on her own coat without help.

At her husband's insistence, she finally agreed to make a doctor's appointment. Right after this, the pain suddenly seemed to have become excruciating. Having finally broken through her denial and acknowledged that something was wrong, Jeanne now felt ten times worse. She realized that she had actually been suppressing the pain, quite unconsciously. She had switched to using her right arm for everything, such as brushing her hair, and she had stopped sleeping on her left side because, as she now realized consciously, lying on her left shoulder was agonizing. Ultimately, an orthopedist diagnosed severe bursitis in Jeanne's shoulder. This healed slowly with rest and medication.

People who are not usually stoical may temporarily minimize symptoms as a result of visiting a doctor whom they trust and believe in. Medical treatment can make you feel better without curing your disease, because the ritual of going to the doctor, the positive expectation that he will be able to help, and the act of undergoing an elaborate, prescribed treatment, all have powerful, nonspecific, beneficial effects. Merely telling your story to an esteemed and trusted professional can be such a relief that you feel physically much better.

People Who Sometimes Feel Sick: The Worried Well

Most of us are neither stoics nor hypochondriacs, but lie somewhere in between. Most of the time we neither amplify nor reduce our bodily sensations. But at particularly difficult times in our lifes, under great stress, we may become a bit hypochondriacal. At such times of crisis, some people go to bed and sleep more, some drink more, some resume cigarette smoking. And many others begin to feel ill and worry about their health. This is a way of reacting to the stress, a way of taking ourselves out of the action temporarily, and this kind of hypochondria subsides when the crisis resolves. People like this have been called "the worried well."

The death of someone important is a good example of such a crisis. It is not uncommon for recently bereaved people to experience bodily symptoms just like those of the person who died, and they may become very frightened, or even convinced, that they have fallen ill with the same disease. A serious, life-threatening illness of your own is another such stress. As we've seen, many patients recovering from heart attacks go through a period during their recuperation when they are obsessed with their health, monitor every trivial bodily sensation, and believe that a medical catastrophe is imminent.

Paula Blackwell's case shows how an average person can experience the vagaries of symptom perception firsthand and gives us a glimpse into what it is like to be among the worried well. Paula is a thirty-three-year-old telephone salesperson whose husband left her suddenly and immediately filed for divorce. She soon learned that he had been carrying on an affair with her cousin for several years, and that he was planning to marry her as soon as possible. Paula was devastated, humiliated, and, later on, infuriated.

Paula has always been healthy, though several of her relatives have died prematurely of heart attacks. She has never thought much about her health and always took her body pretty much for granted. She was a vigorous person and considered herself the farthest thing from a sissy or a complainer. But during a hot spell in July, shortly after her husband had left, it slowly dawned on her that she had been having mild dizzy spells. The next time one occurred, she was quite conscious of it and wondered if it was because she was not getting enough sleep. She lay down to rest. At work three days later, she experienced another episode. This time the room started to spin around her and she really thought she was going to faint. Though she hated complaining to anyone (it seemed childish), she did mention her symptoms to a coworker whose desk was beside hers. Paula's friend thought she should see a doctor right away.

For the first time, Paula became concerned. She began trying to diagnose herself. She compared the vision in her right and left eyes by covering one and then the other, but there seemed to be no difference. She poked her skull to see where it was tender. Though she couldn't find anything wrong, she noticed a visible pulsation over her right temple when she looked in the mirror. And wasn't one corner of her mouth drooping a bit more than the other side? She now became very anxious, and over the next few days the dizziness worsened. Finally, frightened that something serious was wrong, she visited a doctor.

The physician found her in good health. He suggested that Paula's dizziness was due to anxiety and stress. His reassurance promptly halted Paula's worries and her symptoms. On one occasion she thought that she felt dizzy again, but since she no longer feared that she was sick, the symptom was no longer ominous and it slipped from her mind. The whole episode became a thing of the past.

Doctors are just as susceptible as others—perhaps even more so—to this kind of hypochondriacal stress reaction. For example, most medical students have transitory hypochondriacal reactions under the extreme stress of their first intimate contact with desperately ill patients. They become convinced that they have contracted a disease they are studying. Their symptoms often mimic those of one of their patients, perhaps one with whom the student readily identifies because of similarities in age or personal background. The medical student begins to examine himself carefully and perhaps gets a classmate to examine him as well. He then begins visiting the student health service, pleading urgently for the very diagnostic tests he has just been learning about. Eventually he is reassured that he is not in fact mortally ill, and his perception of his body returns to normal.

The cause of medical-student hypochondriasis is a cognitive one. The student mistakenly attributes normal bodily sensations and the symptoms of stress and anxiety to a serious medical disease. In the past the student would have ignored or minimized such symptoms because they weren't significant. But in light of his new body of medical knowledge, these sensations assume a new importance—he knows now that they can be symptoms of serious disorders—and so they alarm him and he focuses upon them and amplifies them.

Sometimes medical-student hypochondriasis can get a little out of hand and even become amusing. One such episode began when a third-year medical student developed back pain and began to worry that he had ruptured a spinal disc.[15] He sought and received a back X ray, shortly after which he began wondering if his testes might have been damaged by radiation exposure during the procedure. He discussed this with the X-ray technician but was not reassured, and so he went to talk with the chief radiologist at the hospital. This conversation only heightened his fears, so he went to the library to survey the literature on accidental irradiation. (His literature review was so meticulous and so exhaustive that the radiologist later found it "acceptable for publication by any journal of radiology.") The student discovered that lead-lined shields were available but not routinely employed by his hospital for this type of X ray. He thereupon drafted a letter, which was signed by a number of his classmates, requesting that such shields be routinely employed in the radiology department. The drama concluded when the students obtained a lead shield from an X-ray supply house and formally presented it to the radiology department.

The elderly are also susceptible to bouts of excessive fright about their health. This may be triggered by the real physical decline and the increasing limitations that accompany aging. Many elderly find it harder to do things that they used to take for granted: hearing deteriorates, climbing stairs becomes more tiring, just getting out of the bathtub may be difficult. The specter of dependency upon others in order to open a door or a can, for help crossing an icy street, arises. Worse yet, old friends and family members die, reminding the elderly person of his own mortality. As physical capacity wanes and infirmities increase, the elderly can find themselves among the worried well—basically healthy, but very worried about disease and disability.

Sometimes it is the loneliness and isolation of the elderly that stimulates a hypochondriacal reaction. For these older persons, it is not so much their physical decline that causes this, but rather it is the need for the interpersonal contact and the basic human attention that accompany medical attention. The visit to the hospital and to the doctor is a major social event for them. They make a day of it, arriving early at the hospital for their appointment in order to sit in the lobby, visit the gift shop to buy a magazine or card, and eat lunch in the cafeteria. For some of these people, the physician is the only human being who physically touches them, and the secretary's call to confirm an appointment may be the only time their telephone rings.

People Who Always Feel Sick: Full-time Hypochondriacs

A hypochondriac is a person who feels ill all the time though he is in fact well. He suffers from the debilitating *idea* that he is sick. And the idea that one is sick can cause invalidism as inexorably as emphysematous lungs or clogged arteries. In *The Guermantes' Way*, by Marcel Proust, a patient taunts his physician: "For each ailment that doctors cure with medications (as I am told they do occasionally succeed in doing), they produce ten others in healthy individuals by inoculating them with that pathogenic agent a thousand times more virulent than all the microbes—the idea that they are ill."[16] The hypochondriac is healthy by objective standards: a careful physical examination discloses no signs of disease, and his laboratory tests are all normal. Yet he believes he is diseased, and he feels ill.

This kind of hypochondriac differs from the worried well people discussed above. He is suffering from a real psychiatric disorder, not a temporary stress reaction. This character is a hypochondriac for life, a person for whom illness and invalidism are a way of life, a way of seeing the world, and a feature of his personality. This is the kind of person who belabors you at a cocktail party with a long and sad monologue about his difficulties, who seems to be endlessly making excuses for himself, and who is only too ready to recount his most recent medical consultation in exquisite detail. If, after five minutes, you try to interject some of your own experiences, you will be met with a blank, uninterested stare, because the hypochondriac seems to be looking more for an audience than a conversation.[17] Almost everyone can reminisce about a hypochondriac like this whom he has known. There always seems to be a cousin with mysterious dizzy spells that could never be diagnosed, or a grandfather who is constantly taking his pulse and examining his throat in the mirror, who irritates the entire family with his self-absorption and his medical excuses.

What Is Hypochondriasis?

Inoculated with the Idea of Illness

Hypochondriasis is a psychiatric disorder characterized by an excessive preoccupation with health, disease, and one's body. The hypochondriac interprets his normal bodily sensations unrealistically, believing that they are a sign of disease. He is afraid of illness, convinced that he is seriously sick. Reassuring him that he is well is of no avail. We are going to discuss the hypochondriac at some length because he has a great deal to tell us about the psychology of health. He can even shed light upon some features of contemporary American culture. Let us start by looking at a typical hypochondriac.

At twenty-nine, Herbert Evans is incapacitated by a puzzling but profound weakness and by headaches and a "post-nasal drip" that have lasted for the past six years. His case is baffling because no one knows what is wrong with Herb; although his symptoms are severe, they have defied the diagnostic efforts of many competent physicians.

Herb has an overwhelming sensation of heaviness in his arms and legs ("It's just like someone had pumped concrete into the center of my bones"), and he almost always feels ill in one way or another. Many symptoms have bedeviled him over the years, including a feeling that his head is too full and "cloudy," constipation, a "drawing" pain in his chest, and dizziness. On the days when Herb doesn't feel sick, he worries that whatever he wants to do (like staying out late at a jazz concert) will somehow overtax him and make him ill again. Most often, he just feels too sick to concentrate at work, to have a social life, or to complete any do-it-yourself projects around the house. He likens himself to his favorite basketball team, whose exhaustion at the end of a draining season caused them to lose their concentration, make "mental errors," and falter in the playoffs.

All of Herb's laboratory tests and physical examinations have been completely normal; to judge him by these objective measures, he is a young man in perfect health. But his symptoms persist, and so he has grown increasingly frustrated with his physicians and their smug assurances that "nothing is wrong." For this is certainly not true from his perspective—something most definitely is wrong.

This young man's troubles began with his first job as a reporter for a prestigious newspaper after finishing journalism school, when it soon became apparent that his career would not be the meteoric one he and his father, a famous newspaper editor, had hoped for. His work was not well received, and soon his symptoms began. This was also soon after he had married a young woman he had met while vacationing in Florida. His wife, ambitious and bright, went on rapidly to become an assistant producer at a local television station. Herb became increasingly reproachful because it didn't seem to him that she was understanding enough about his illness or supportive enough of him. Instead, she seemed to be growing less sympathetic, and now at times she implied that he was a hypochondriac. He had originally expected to have children, but when the time came, he felt that raising children would be too demanding and only make him feel sicker.

Herb had always been a sports enthusiast, but even this withered away in the shadow cast by his illness. Though a basketball star in high school and college, he had had to stop playing on his newspaper's basketball team because it seemed that his sore throats were particularly likely to recur the day after a strenuous game. For a while he continued to be an avid fan of professional sports and attended many games in person. But with time he was reduced to watching his favorite teams on television, lying on the sofa, often in his bathrobe.

As Herb saw it, he was an invalid, crippled by a disease that had sapped his strength and promise, ruined his career, and taken its toll on his marriage. He felt "like a boxer hanging on for the bell," struggling to lose a match on his feet rather than knocked out flat on his back. His only source of pride was his perserverence, his refusal to give up in the face of his affliction.

His own peculiar curse, the thing that made his affliction so uniquely awful, was that there was no diagnosis, no label, no explanation that would at least legitimize his symptoms in the eyes of others. Receiving a diagnosis, he felt, would at least remove the aspersion that nothing was really wrong with him, that he was making it all up, that it was all in his head. Hence a diagnosis became his Holy Grail. He persistently sought medical attention, running a gauntlet of subspecialists whom he besought to repeat laboratory tests that had already been normal many times. He kept a detailed diary of his symptoms and was followed simultaneously by physicians at four different hospitals. He read extensively in medical texts, compiling his own list of possible diagnoses. Yet Herb found no relief, or even any satisfactory explanation, and went on like this for years. He illustrates the important features of hypochondriasis: bodily symptoms that can't be explained medically, the belief that one is gravely ill, a preoccupation with health, and unhappy relationships with doctors.

Hypochondriacal Bodily Symptoms

People like Herb Evans can have terrible symptoms that torment and cripple them but have no medical basis. Many hypochondriacal complaints are similar to normal bodily sensations that most of us disregard. Sometimes, though, the symptoms are unusual and highly personalized, such as "My veins ache," "One leg weighs more than the other," "I have dry ears" or "sleepy hands." The symptoms are described imprecisely, so that it is very difficult for the doctor to obtain a clear history. For example, the response to the question "Is the headache worse in the morning?" may be "Yes, and it's worse in the afternoon too." When the doctor asks, "How many times have you had it?," the hypochondriac answers, "All the time."

In contrast to this vague description of what he is feeling, the hypochondriac has a vivid and elaborate notion of what is going on inside his body to cause the symptom. As one patient wrote in a long letter to her internist, "In the abdomen it feels like an internal pulling and stretching. When I sit or lie down, this internal stress starts immediately. Frequently in this area, I feel the stress of something blowing up like a balloon to a point where I feel it should burst. There is no relief of these conditions until I stand up." Like Mr. Evans, the hypochondriac is usually very concerned with the meaning and authenticity of his symptoms. Sometimes this troubles him as much as the discomfort itself, and so he seeks a diagnosis and an explanation as much as symptom relief.

Attitudes and Beliefs About Disease

Once certain fears and beliefs about disease take hold, you feel sick even when you aren't. Hypochondriasis is fundamentally a belief system. The hypochondriac has a profound and unshakable conviction that he has an undetected, serious disease. Neither repeated reassurance from doctors nor negative physical examinations nor a benign course over time allays his conviction. This contrasts with the worried well patient who feels much better after receiving appropriate reassurance. Over the years, Mr. Evans remained unwavering in his belief that he harbored an occult disease, and he hoped if he went to enough physicians and had enough tests performed, eventually a diagnosis would be made. The hypochondriac's conviction is so strong that he adamantly and angrily rejects any suggestion that nonmedical factors such as life stress or emotions might play a role in his suffering. (In contrast, patients with actual medical disorders are often willing to entertain the possibility that psychological factors have played some role in their getting sick or in making their illness worse.)

Hypochondriacs are also afraid, terrified of disease. The slightest hint of illness is cause for alarm, for example, reading about a disease or hearing about someone who became sick. Common, benign sensations are a source of consternation: a gas pain is interpreted as angina pectoris, a freckle becomes skin cancer. The hypochondriac's sense that he is about to receive a death sentence is anguishing. As Sir

William Petty said in a letter to the famous seventeenth-century British chemist Robert Boyle (who was a hypochondriac), "The . . . disease you labor under, is your apprehension of many diseases, and a continual fear that you are inclining or falling into one or other. Here I might tell you the vanity of life; or, that to fear any evil long is more intolerable than the evil itself suffered."[18]

The Preoccupation with Health and One's Body

Healthy people can become more preoccupied with their bodies and their symptoms than people with serious diseases, as the hypochondriac, in his obsession with his body, demonstrates. Normal physiological functions fascinate him endlessly, and he carries out elaborate self-diagnosis and self-treatment rituals. His interpersonal relationships are dominated by health concerns, and he discusses his symptoms at length with others, complaining vociferously and quite publicly of his plight. Physical symptoms become a vocabulary for relating to other people, a way to communicate where words fail. He strikes up friendships with others because they have a same doctor or the same symptom, and hours are passed recounting medical histories and comparing medications.

The hypochondriac's health is thus a key part of his identity. He is no longer *afflicted* with his symptoms, he has *become* his symptoms. Like Mr. Evans, the only things he takes pride in are his ability to endure physical suffering, his fortitude in the face of great hardship, and the simple fact that he has managed to survive.

Hypochondriacs and Doctors

Our medical-care system does not do well by healthy people who feel ill. When bodily complaints do not result from a medical disorder, medical diagnosis and medical treatment are not helpful. In most doctors' minds, symptoms reflect an underlying disease, and their job is to decode the symptoms to disclose the disease causing them. But symptomatic patients who are "well" don't fit into this medical model. Unable to diagnose a disease, the doctor can offer no cure.

Hypochondriacs thus fall into a peculiar no-man's land between medicine and psychiatry. They gravitate to medical settings since they feel medically ill. Yet internal-medicine specialists can't treat them because they find no disease. Psychiatrists are more interested in the condition but rarely encounter hypochondriacs in mental-health settings.

Hypochondriacs are very trying to take care of, and they present a characteristic picture in the doctor's office. They arrive with long symptom diaries, lists of all the medications they have ever taken and their side effects, and their old medical records and X rays. They immediately launch into a difficult-to-interrupt, extensive litany of symptoms, sometimes referred to as an "organ recital." They frequently telephone their doctors between appointments, and their seemingly endless complaints and insatiable neediness sometimes cause doctors to think of them as "black holes." One hospitalized patient, for example, had her doctor paged while he was still at the nursing station outside her room, having just left her bedside. She wanted a Band-Aid.

Yet the hypochondriac feels profoundly ambivalent toward doctors; as much as he needs them, he demeans and devalues them at the same time. The patient spurns the doctor's attempts to be helpful, disparages his abilities, and tells him he is making things worse, with hostility that is barely concealed.

For their part, most physicians also regard hypochondriacs with ambivalence. The hypochondriac gets under the physician's skin because, on the one hand, he is demanding and clinging, while on the other he is angry and hostile. As much as the doctor wants to be helpful and tries to be helpful, nothing works. Indeed, the patient seems almost hellbent on defeating his efforts: most of the doctor's interventions produce either complications, disturbing side effects, or new symptoms to replace the old ones. His frustration is of course compounded when his patient keeps returning, ungrateful. The physician may begin to feel that he has other, "sicker," patients for whom his skill is better employed. Hypochondriacs can be so burdensome and unpleasant, and caring for them can be so taxing and vexing, that the doctor may even wish he were rid of them (though few go as far as one physician who offered to pay his patient to go to a different doctor). Sometimes, in their frustration, doctors call hypochondriacs "trolls," "gomers" (an acronym for Get Out of My Emergency Room), and "turkeys." Hospital emergency rooms have been known to harbor signs in the format of the standard international road sign, with a large red circle with a red line through the black silhouette of a turkey. Because they are also often called "crocks," their care is referred to as "psychoceramic medicine," and the appropriate diagnostic test is termed the "serum porcelain level."

So while doctors' visits and medical examinations are a way of life for the hypochondriac, his medical care is as unsatisfactory as it is extensive.

In Summary

When it comes to feeling sick, things may not be as they seem: having symptoms does not necessarily mean that we have a disease. Our perception of what is going on inside our bodies is often unreliable. The hypochondriac is a vivid illustration of how far illness and disease can diverge. But this phenomenon is not limited to the experience of chronic hypochondriacs. Old age and social isolation tend to bring out worries about health, as do certain personality traits, such as being introspective and self-aware, or feeling that we have little control over what happens to us in life. Many of us mislead ourselves about our health at various times: when we are healthy but under stress and develop disturbing symptoms; when we have a serious medical illness but our fears make us feel far sicker; when we go to a doctor and his reassurance that we are well relieves troublesome but benign symptoms. And most important, the belief that we are sick, the fear of disease, and the preoccupation with our bodies can in themselves disable us and make us into invalids.

CHAPTER 4

Why People Feel Sick

WE HAVE DISCUSSED *how* we perceive the symptoms of ill health, and *who* tends to feel sicker. In this chapter we will explain *why* we sometimes feel sicker than we really are. There are a number of reasons: illness is a nonverbal way of asking for affection; our becoming a patient is rewarded by family members or provides a way out of a difficult life situation; the body can be a metaphor for expressing how we feel about ourselves as persons; and the culture around us amplifies our private health concerns and minor health problems and makes them seem worse.

We will be using the term *functional* to describe some symptoms. It refers to symptoms for which there is no adequate medical basis or explanation. They are contrasted with "organic symptoms," which are symptoms that can be accounted for on the basis of a known disease or disease mechanism.

A Bodily Pantomime

We all need an audience with whom we can share our feelings and our concerns. Physical distress may be embraced because it gathers that audience around us, because it elicits an exceptional dose of sympathy, support, and assistance. To tell someone about your aches and pains is to ask him for help; disclosing your suffering brings people to your side. For some, the resulting encouragement and attention substitute for the real affection and genuine love that is lacking in their lives. Pain and illness thus help them to feel that they are cared about and looked after. Such people don't express their neediness in so many words but have unconsciously discovered that they can ask for kindness and special consideration covertly—by feeling ill. They are saying with their symptoms, "If you can't love me, then at least take care of me."

Functional symptoms can thus be unconscious attempts to reopen broken channels of communication, to tell someone important that something has gone wrong in our lives, and to ask for their help. The sufferer quite unconsciously finds himself using symptoms to communicate where words fail, enacting a kind of bodily pantomime. He is saying, "I am suffering. Please take care of me and be especially considerate now that I am hurt." This mechanism is thought to be important in hypochondriasis, because it has been observed that most hypochondriacal symptoms are addressed *to* someone; were the hypochondriac to land on a desert island, his pains would disappear.[1]

We learn this lesson that pain brings love in infancy. A baby cries when he is hungry, colicky, or hurt when he falls. His lament brings his mother immediately to his side and she bathes him in affection and assuages his suffering. Such childhood experiences teach us to amplify physical suffering in later life when we need love and assistance. We are saying with our symptoms, "Treat me like when I had the mumps."[2]

Some children, in fact, only know tenderness, gentleness, and affection when they are ailing. One young woman, for example, fondly recalled a hospitalization for a tonsillectomy when she was eleven, because her illness had brought her a rare moment of closeness with her mother. She treasured her mother's driving her to the hospital for the surgery because it was the only time she ever remembered having her mother all to herself in the car, without having any other siblings along. Other children grow up with a chronically ill sibling who corners the lion's share of the family's attention. So when they hurt emotionally in later life, as adults, they cry out in physical pain, hoping to obtain the same portion of love, attention, and sympathy.

Edith Mathews is a seventy-seven-year-old healthy grandmother whose story shows us how we use symptoms to tell the important people in our lives that something has gone wrong and to ask their help. Edith's social network has been shrinking. Her husband succumbed suddenly to a heart attack six years ago, and in the last three years she has attended the funerals of two sisters and her closest friend. The most important people in her life right now are her two young grandchildren, who live twenty minutes away, and Edith tries to take them out for pizza every few weeks. She spends much of her time knitting clothes and making gifts for them. But her son-in-law has found a more promising job in a southern city that is more than four hours away by car, and Edith gave up driving several years ago because of cataracts. Suddenly she is confronted with the devastating prospect of losing the only important people in her life.

Edith begins to feel weaker and she thinks her vision is worsening. She goes out less and less. She gets anxious at night, feels short of breath, and worries that if she has a heart attack, there will be no one to help her. She calls her daughter one night complaining of breathlessness. Yet when her daughter arrives, she finds that giving Edith some cocoa and putting her to bed is all that is needed. In calling for help, Edith is asking her family not to desert her. Not surprisingly, her symptoms subside when it is decided that she should move with her family to their new home.

Expressing Anger and Hostility

Some people suffer with functional symptoms because this allows them to express hostile and aggressive feelings in a subtle but effective way. They transform *reproach toward others* into *complaints to* others.[3] First, by displaying their suffering and misery, they arouse the other person's sympathy and elicit a desire to help. But then they thwart the person's assistance, dismissing it as ineffective and inadequate. They complain that their suffering is no better or has actually worsened, subtly implying that the Good Samaritan is a bungler who has only made matters worse. Those around the sufferer, including physicians and family, end up feeling impotent and guilty, wondering if they were responsible for the misery in the first place.

The sufferer's anger may originate in past disappointments, rejections, and losses that came at the hands of caretakers earlier in life (most often parents). These past frustrations are expressed in the present in an unconscious attempt to get back at those who originally let him down. When people in our current life don't seem loyal enough or helpful enough, when they don't live up to our expectations, when they disappoint us by being too absorbed in their own problems and uninterested in ours, we may unconsciously express our anger and frustration as bodily distress.[4]

Doctors often encounter anger in the help-rejecting behavior of patients with severe functional symptoms. For example, a woman complained at length to a consulting psychiatrist about her multiple physical symptoms, which she felt had been inadequately treated by her previous physicians. She was desperate for help and asked the psychiatrist for the name of a specialist whom she might consult. When given a name, she sniffed that she had never heard it before and so suspected the doctor was not experienced enough to unravel her "complex" case. She then asked the psychiatrist to treat her "nervous stomach" with a tranquilizer. He gave her a prescription, but she reported at the next visit that she had never filled it because she had decided that it would not have worked. Later she asked him to refer her to a stress-reduction program. He spent a considerable amount of time locating a suitable program. But when he called the patient back with the referral, she informed him that she had changed her mind. This patient's anger stemmed from feeling that her husband was not responsive enough or solicitous enough of her. But she found it safer to vent this resentment on her doctors, belaboring them with her complaints and foiling their attempts to treat them at the same time.

Families Can Encourage Symptoms

As was hinted at in the preceding sections, a family's response to a member's complaints influences how sick he feels, what he thinks about his symptoms, and how disabled he becomes. In short, families can encourage or discourage bodily distress and suffering. When a wife asks her husband whether she should call in sick for work, he can shape her experience of illness depending upon whether he brings breakfast to her in bed and offers to call her boss for her, or stalks out muttering that she is just feeling sorry for herself. When we talk about our symptoms, and when we show our distress by taking medicine, lying down, limping, or wincing, we elicit very definite responses from our relatives. Families may respond to a member's suffering by becoming oversolicitous or by ignoring him. These responses variously affect how ill we feel. Somatic symptoms, no matter what their cause, have a way of lingering and worsening when the family responds positively to them.

Though the sick person may at first glance seem to be the weakest and most defenseless member of the family, he is often in fact the most powerful member, because his illness entitles him to special consideration, and his needs now have top priority: a sick family member can cause routine family life to grind to a halt and center on him. Think of the family's response to a sick child. His favorite foods are cooked on demand, and we buy him new toys to occupy his time. Siblings have to watch the television programs he chooses, and if he gives them a hard time, *they* are reprimanded. In addition, the sick member of a family can say and do things that he wouldn't be allowed to get away with otherwise. He can, as we've seen, use his symptoms as an excuse to express anger at other family members (temper outbursts are excusable if you are ill), or use them to avoid sexual intimacy ("not tonight, dear, I have a headache").

Because illness confers such power, it can sometimes be a solution to family problems. One member's illness may reduce friction and lower the overall level of tension within the family as a whole, especially if it distracts everyone else from their interpersonal conflicts by causing them to focus on the identified patient.[5] (We see the same thing among nations, when, for example, the antipathies between the United States and Soviet Union were laid aside temporarily while they became allies against the Nazis.) Thus, as her parents' marriage comes apart, a thirteen-year-old girl may develop tension headaches if these distract her parents and halt their arguments while they unite in trying to make her more comfortable. The result reinforces the child's symptoms, for she has accomplished something that she could not in any other way.

When a patient's suffering stabilizes an otherwise highly unstable family situation, then his symptoms may far exceed whatever medical disease he may have. This seems to happen most in families that are rigid, enmeshed, and unable to acknowledge their difficulties openly.[6] The following story illustrates this. Louisa Wagner is a forty-seven-year-old housewife and mother of three grown children. She has rheumatoid arthritis, which has been treated with aspirin and other painkillers. Though her doctor could find no evidence that her arthritis was actually getting worse, over the course of six months Louisa reported steadily increasing pain, stiffness, and disability. During this period, her youngest son, Jeff, got divorced and moved back to live with his parents. Jeff and Louisa's husband never got along, and now they were almost always arguing. This disturbed Mrs. Wagner a great deal, especially since her own father had had violent fights with her brother when she was growing up.

When her arthritis symptoms worsened, her husband spent more of his time with her, drove her everywhere, and took over the housekeeping. This left him less time and energy to battle with his son. Thus Mrs. Wagner's illness called a truce in the family. When Jeff finally moved out of the house, her symptoms declined to previous levels.

Sickness as the Solution to a Problem

We tend to think of being sick as an unmitigated disaster: painful, frightening, disruptive, costly. But there is another side to it: being ill and being a patient have some compensations. We have already discussed several that may come from one's family. But more generally, being sick can get us out of sticky life situations, providing a solution to various problems.

We can appreciate the compensations inherent in sickness by recognizing that the sick have a unique role, termed by sociologists the sick role, which has its own set of tangible benefits and privileges. The sick person is excused from certain obligations of daily life, from taking out the garbage to cooking the meals. He can postpone challenges he may be facing, such as asking his employer for a raise or meeting a deadline. He can avoid responsibilities, such as going to work or taking an examination. And the sick role may even include financial rewards such as disability payments or insurance awards. On top of everything else, since you are not held responsible for getting sick in the first place, since it is not your *fault* that you are ill, there is no blame or implication of failure in relinquishing your duties and responsibilities.

But you cannot assume the sick role just by claiming it unilaterally. You must be admitted to the sick role by a doctor, who confers that special status upon you by certifying that you have a disease (giving you a diagnosis), and by placing you under his care. In other words, the criteria for admission to the sick role are, first, a diagnosable disease, and second, a good-faith attempt to get better, which you make by placing yourself under the ongoing care of a doctor.

Some hypochondriacs and people with functional symptoms can be understood when we see them as people who seek the sick role but who lack the admission criterion, namely, a medical disease. This explains why the hypochondriac pursues a diagnosis so fervently and is so passionately concerned with the authenticity of his symptoms. To be accorded the sick role, he must be known to have a disease, hence his characteristic disappointment when diagnostic tests are negative, and his sense of vindication if he finally receives some sort of diagnostic label from a physician. However, the doctor's attempts at treatment are unwelcome and threatening, since they foreshadow future dismissal from the sick role when the symptoms have been cured. The patient therefore counters with more severe symptoms, side effects of the treatment, or entirely new complaints to replace the old ones.

When we talk about "seeking" the sick role, it is important to reemphasize that such behavior is unconscious and the sufferers are not feigning or simulating illness. They are indeed experiencing the bodily discomfort they describe and simply remain unaware of the emotional and psychological basis for their symptoms.

Turning Sentiment into Sensation

We feel emotion in our bodies. We "burn" with anger, "tremble" with fear, feel "choked up" with sadness; our "stomachs turn" with revulsion. Everyone tends to experience unpleasant emotions as unpleasant bodily sensations and thus to feel physically distressed when emotionally distressed. This tendency to distract ourselves with physical sensation is called somatization, which is the selective focus on the bodily symptoms of psychological distress while minimizing the mental and emotional aspects of the distress. Examples like this one abound: after an argument with your landlord, you are more aware of a pounding headache than of your fury.

We are taught to somatize as we grow up. We learn it from friends and schoolmates, from neighbors and parents. Siblings teach by example: if a young sister is excused from having to eat her vegetables at dinner because of a stomach ache, it will not be long before her brother who hates milk will develop a similar complaint.

The child who is emotionally upset and the child who is physically ill may both report the same feelings: a generalized complaint that they simply do not feel right. Sick children can't describe their condition precisely, can't tell us just what bodily symptoms they have or where in their bodies they feel them. Illness to a child is a global concept, encompassing emotions, moods, physical distress, and the inability to engage in desired activities. Young children define healthiness as being able to do the things they wish and feeling happy and good in general. Thus parents often note as the first sign of medical illness a change in the child's behavior—apathy or lack of energy, for example.

As he grows, the child is taught how to assess different states of distress and how to describe them. He learns which sensations are part of an emotion and which are labeled as bodily symptoms. If his family ignores or explicitly devalues open and direct emotional display but responds positively to physical distress, the child learns to somatize. If complaints of a sore throat result in mother's consent to stay home from school while complaints that he is unhappy do not, then the child is taught to focus on the bodily sensations of emotion and to minimize the sentiments themselves. And this is generally the case, because if psychological symptoms confer patienthood at all, they do it less honorably than do physical symptoms.

Some studies seem to confirm this observation by finding that parental overattentiveness to children's physical complaints produces adults who have more minor and transient bodily symptoms. Researchers have found that adults who are high symptom reporters had mothers who were more likely to keep them home from school because of illness and who were more symptomatic themselves.[7] Other studies, however, have failed to confirm such a relationship.

Having been taught to somatize, as adults we all do it to some degree, with the result that we may feel quite sick physically when we really are not. Think of an ambiguous symptom such as loss of appetite. Do we ascribe it to a mild, lingering flu or to our anxiety over an upcoming meeting with the boss? Depression is often somatized, since it has both physical and emotional components. Severely depressed people feel sad, guilty, self-critical, and hopeless. But somatic symptoms are also part of the depressive disorder: fatigue, loss of appetite, insomnia, constipation, among other things. The depressed person may focus upon either constellation of symptoms.

Culture influences our tendency to somatize. Depression serves as an example. Severely depressed people the world over suffer with the same physical and mental symptoms, but they describe their illness in very different terms. In most cultures, depressed patients do not report emotional or cognitive symptoms at all and instead complain exclusively of aches and pains. For instance, in China, fatigue is a common psychiatric diagnosis, while depression is hardly diagnosed there at all. Chinese patients complain of headaches, insomnia, and pain, along with their fatigue, but only 9 percent of them admit feeling sad or guilty or hopeless. Yet when these patients are carefully examined by Western psychiatrists, 87 percent of them are diagnosed as being seriously depressed.[8] From our American viewpoint, the Chinese suppress the emotional symptoms of depression and focus instead upon its somatic symptoms.

Language is one way in which different cultures shape the perception and expression of bodily distress. You can't complain of a feeling that you don't have a word for. Cultures evolve many different words to denote fine distinctions between those conditions that are particularly important to them.[9] Thus languages vary in the number and specificity of words they contain for describing emotions and internal bodily states. For example, our language distinguishes among anger, hostility, and resentment, and among sadness, despondency, and demoralization. In contrast, there are African languages with a single word that refers to both anger and sadness.

It is not hard to see that children growing up in different cultural traditions would learn to express their physical distress in alternative ways. People from backgrounds in which it is acceptable to express emotional distress do so more readily than people from backgrounds in which it is considered shameful and is discouraged and deprecated.

Narcissism
The Narcissistic Personality

People can feel sicker than they really are because their feelings about their bodies sometimes symbolize the way they think about themselves as people. In other words, their feelings about their bodies are a metaphor for their feelings about themselves.

The concept of narcissism is relevant here. Narcissism is the love of oneself, the excitement and gratification that come from admiring oneself and one's physical and mental attributes. It is our pride, our self-esteem, our positive self-regard. The word *narcissism,* in fact, is derived from Narcissus, the mythological figure who fell in love with his own reflected image.

Narcissism is normal in young children and persists in diluted form in psychologically healthy adults. As long as it is kept in proper perspective, it is a valuable ingredient of the mature personality: we all need a healthy dose of self-esteem and self-confidence, a basic acceptance of who we are and a pride in our assets. Well-integrated narcissism is necessary for a sense of security and well-being, for a basic feeling of self-respect and of being at peace with ourselves. It allows us to derive pleasure from our gifts and abilities, and it provides us with an appropriate feeling of being valuable, worthwhile, and special. It is this healthy narcissism that also calms and soothes each of us in times of rejection and failure.

But if narcissism persists into adulthood in an unrealistic or exaggerated form, it can produce disturbing, even incapacitating, psychological problems. When someone is vain and self-centered, when he acts as if we ought to pay for the privilege of even knowing him, we call him narcissistic in this pathological sense. But his smugness and superior air actually conceal a deeper view of himself that is quite the opposite—a private sense of himself as defective, inferior, empty, and worthless. His external conceit and egotism, his apparent self-satisfaction, mask a painfully fragile sense of self-esteem.

The narcissist oscillates between two extremes, superiority and inferiority. He may be intoxicated with how superior and unique he is at one moment, but his exquisite sensitivity to failure and slights makes him vulnerable to profound shame, embarrassment, and humiliation a minute later. The giddy flush of elation that follows a compliment from someone evaporates as soon as the other person ceases paying tribute. A young man is ecstatic when his beautiful date tells him how attractive he looks, but he is crushed minutes later when she fails to comment on his expensive sports car.

Lacking a solid inner sense of who he is, what he does well and what he does poorly, what his strengths and weaknesses are, the narcissist concentrates on his external image. The surface, the envelope, the external impression is so crucial because everything inside seems flimsy and precarious. The narcissist must have the "right" look, the "right" car, the "right" address. When he shops for clothes, for example, he does not even know what he himself prefers, but can think only in terms of what other people will perceive as the right image. Because external appearances are so critical, the narcissist stresses physical beauty, sexual prowess (sexual *performance* being more important than sexual *feelings*), and physical strength. His body is one of his most precious and cherished possessions. He may work out constantly and become totally absorbed in how he looks from every angle. Yet when he sees himself in the mirror, he instantly zeroes in on any blemishes and flaws, however minor. Unattractive features and imperfections, such as large feet or heavy eyebrows, are almost impossible to ignore or to accept.

When viewed from the outside, the narcissist may appear free of psychological problems and seem to be an effective, charming, and "together" person. He may indeed, to return to the example above, choose beautiful clothes and look wonderful. But the problem is on the inside: his clothes do not express his taste, or how he feels about himself, but are only part of a calculated performance, a mask. One young woman expressed this, remarking that "I feel like a compliment that I'm beautiful is just a compliment to my makeup." Beneath the surface, the narcissist feels inauthentic, false, and shallow, and his life seems to have no durable meaning or significance. At work, for all his superficial success, he does not experience himself as truly skillful or competent, but feels that he is just acting as if he were.

Since the narcissist lacks a solid sense of self-esteem, he is, as we've noted, exquisitely sensitive to the feedback from those around him. He must continually prop up his precarious sense of himself by impressing other people and then basking in the glow of their admiration. In effect, he is reduced to constantly asking "How am I doing?" Thus it is not surprising that narcissists often gravitate to fields in which there is a chance of receiving adulation and worship, such as the theater, athletics, politics, or academics. The narcissist is an exhibitionist because of his continual need to be applauded, envied, and idolized.

On the other hand, since his inner sense of himself is so

rickety, the narcissist is painfully sensitive to failure. Because his ambitions are so great, there is greater room for failure. Every disappointment is a devastating defeat, making him feel totally unworthy, defective, and utterly inadequate. Personal setbacks feel like wounds that are deliberately inflicted on him by someone else, and the narcissist reacts not with feelings of sadness or loss, but rather with rage, resentment, and the desire for revenge.

In his dealings with other people, the narcissist is egotistical and selfish. Being profoundly self-centered, he tends to manipulate, intimidate, seduce, and exploit others for his benefit. His interpersonal relationships are shallow because he is not genuinely interested in the other person but is merely using him like a mirror, for self-enhancement. So the narcissist is often drawn to especially beautiful members of the opposite sex. He only mimics caring about them, though, since his primary object of devotion is himself.

Narcissism and the Perception of Health

The use of the body as a metaphor for the psyche is perfectly normal and occurs in us all. If you feel "weak" because you didn't ask your boss for the raise you want, you may end up feeling physically weak and fatigued. When your self-esteem is wounded because none of your coworkers asked you to lunch with them, you may end up feeling unattractive or worrying that your new haircut makes you look foolish. Your body becomes a symbol for expressing how you feel about yourself psychologically.

But this happens excessively in the narcissist, who feels frail and fragile *as a person* but expresses that feeling by viewing *his body* in that way. The following story shows how bodily discomfort can express the narcissist's psychological discomfort. A successful computer-software entrepreneur, Steve Morosco was "shattered" after a relatively minor business deal foundered. Although his firm's overall position was not threatened, Steve felt totally humiliated and was haunted by the idea that his "image as a winner" had been destroyed.

Beneath his outwardly assured and smooth manner, Steve harbored profound doubts about himself. He had always suspected that his successes were due to good luck rather than ability, and this one failure punctured his veneer of self-confidence and deflated him like a balloon. He now suddenly saw himself as "a total loser." He worried that his career had lost its "momentum," that his "winning record" was fatally blemished. It seemed that all his peers were going places, while he, by contrast, was only marking time, treading water. He became frightened that he would rapidly be surpassed by his competitors; when he saw one of them on the street with a beautiful woman he himself had dated once, Steve had a panic attack. He developed episodes of breathlessness, sweating, and feeling faint, and he complained of ringing in his ears. His body felt insubstantial, as if it were made of papier-mâché, and he complained that vibrations in the environment, such as those resulting from central air conditioning, made his internal organs tremble.

Everyone becomes depressed and angry at a business setback, but Steve was devastated by a relatively minor one because he was so narcissistic, his supremely self-confident veneer never having been backed up by a deep-seated feeling that he was strong enough to weather defeats and losses. Steve saw no link between his setback at work and his somatic symptoms, though he described his physical and psychological well-being in similar terms: he felt emotionally disoriented, thrown off stride, and he noted that he felt unstable when walking and kept losing his balance; he felt psychologically shattered by his setback, and he described his health as "shattered" also. During psychotherapy, Steve gained a more solid, durable, and realistic sense of himself. Once he did this, he was able to put the upsetting events into perspective; he felt less shaken by what had happened. He was able to get back on his feet and resume his career. His medical symptoms and health concerns gradually lessened.

Because the narcissist does not experience himself or, by extension, his body as vital or sound or solid, he is terrified of disease and infirmity, since it seems as if these could easily befall him. He may feel so physically vulnerable that he becomes overly afraid of being assaulted on the street or of being injured in physical activities, such as hiking in the woods.

We've all had the experience of "losing our cool": perhaps we made a stupid remark when out to dinner with friends, and we suddenly felt self-conscious, awkward, and clumsy for a while as we ate and drank. But the narcissist takes the psychological hurt further, totally losing the sense of his body as a strong, healthy, integrated whole. He worries that his health and his body are deteriorating, and he feels sick and enfeebled.

Narcissists also have a special terror of aging and physical decline. Catherine Black, for example, was a physician who sought medical attention for a tremor in her hands shortly after her sixty-second birthday. She had had the tremor for her entire life and had never sought treatment for it before, as it was barely noticeable and had not worsened. But now it tormented her.

Dr. Black had recently begun to feel old and unattractive, and hearing herself speaking in a store one day, she was shocked to note that it was the voice of an old woman. The experience of aging is painful for many, but it was so humiliating for Dr. Black that she became obsessed with a barely detectable symptom. Her inability to control the movement of her hands seemed in her mind to symbolize her growing old. She was haunted by the fear that others would notice her tremor and view her as aged and declining. She therefore began to eat alone as much as possible, and though an accomplished flutist, she ceased playing with her chamber music group.

Dr. Black found aging so anguishing because of the kind of person she is. As she talked at length to her doctor about what she was going through, she realized that she was most unhappy about growing old because it meant she was never going to realize her secret fantasies of unlimited success, wealth, and power. She had harbored secret, lifelong dreams of great political success. Now it hit her that this was not to be.

As a young woman she had attended a top women's college and a prestigious medical school. It had seemed that there were no limits to what she could accomplish in life. She had never married because she felt it would undermine her professional ambitions. Indeed, her professional success brought esteem from her colleagues, admiration from her students, and the adoration of her patients. And if in the back of her mind it all fell short of being a congresswoman or a mayor, still, the future lay ahead. Now that it had finally hit her that her political ambitions would go unfulfilled, she became fixated upon tangible symbols of her disappointment: her trembling hands, the change in the quality of her voice, the loss of vigor in her step.

The bodily signs of maturity horrify the narcissist because beauty, celebrity, physical prowess, and power—the qualities that he prizes and with which he garners admiration—decline with age. In confronting the prospect of their own deaths, many people find some consolation in old friendships, in a commitment to some past achievements or personal values, in a continuing intellectual interest in the world. But these are of little comfort to the narcissist.

The Public Psychology of Health

A cultural climate of alarm about health can heighten each individual's feelings of ill-health and foster a personal sense of dis-ease. The contemporary culture furnishes a context, a health ideology, and an emotional atmosphere that affect each of us personally. Cultural values, norms, and attitudes influence private feelings of healthiness through the four amplifiers we discussed in chapter 2: attention, beliefs, circumstances, and moods. Through them, a societal preoccupation with health and medical care nurtures an insecure public, disturbed by our frailties and ailments, increasingly worried about our health.

The description of Frank Carson with which we opened the book is also a description of contemporary America. Frank was swept up in an avalanche of messages about health: radio advertisements, mail solicitations, casual conversations, a luncheon menu, a store display, a newspaper column. Our society's heightened health consciousness prompts all of us to concentrate more on our own health, to pore over our bodies and our every sensation, just as Frank did. And the more we scrutinize ourselves, the more things we find wrong with us. This constant focusing of attention on our health then makes our symptoms seem worse and makes us feel more ill. We constantly read and hear of the health hazards lurking in our lifestyles, diet, and environment, of the continual need for medical care. This climate of unease, fueled by pervasive health reportage, provides an ominous and worrisome context that can amplify everyday ailments and minor symptoms. Our culture also provides a multitude of disease attributions for every benign bodily sensation. The message is that every symptom, no matter how innocent, must be taken seriously because it might portend grave illness. This doctrine contributes to a declining collective sense of healthiness and physical well-being, for the more diseases we hear about, the more diseases we imagine we have.

There is also an increasing social sanction of health-related behavior. The quest for a healthy lifestyle is widely approved. Under this socially acceptable guise, people with hypochondriacal tendencies may gratify them through exercise fanaticism, stringent and extreme diets, elaborate rituals to protect themselves from environmental health hazards, do-it-yourself diagnostic kits, and strenuous efforts to educate themselves about health and medicine. While we do not applaud the dinner party guest who recounts his history of gallstones throughout the meal, it is perfectly acceptable dinner conversation for joggers to discuss their resting pulse rates, the state of their ankles, and the virtues of high-protein diets. And while ten years ago we might have labeled tales of lethal tap water paranoid, it is now perfectly acceptable to refuse anything but bottled water.

Medication Doesn't Cure the Need to Be Sick

Though Frank Carson was healthy, he lacked a feeling of physical well-being. His attempts to take care of himself led not to enhanced feelings of healthiness but instead to further apprehension and insecurity and dis-ease. Frank lives in a society that may have reached a similar point of diminishing returns. Many healthy Americans are worried about their bodies and their health. How have we arrived at this point, and where will it lead?

A feeling of healthiness requires more than being bio-chemically and physiologically normal. It depends upon our view of ourselves as people, upon our emotional content-ment, and upon the state of our personal relationships. People may feel sicker than they really are when they displace feelings about themselves onto their bodies; when they sub-stitute physical pain for emotional pain; when they use the language of illness to say something to someone; when ill-ness brings personal and family rewards that can't be ob-tained in any other way; and when the society around them nurtures their health concerns.

To the degree that bodily distress stems from psychologi-cal and interpersonal distress, medical care will fail to make us feel better. For "there is no medication that will alter the psychological need for illness, and no surgical procedure that will cut it out." This is what physicians discover as they toil fruitlessly with their hypochondriacal patients. And it is what their patients discover when all the examinations and laboratory tests and prescriptions fail to bring relief. Again, the logic may extend to our society as a whole. If our heightened health consciousness is fueled by underlying psychological and social concerns, then working out, dieting, reading up on medicine, and all of our other health-conscious pursuits will not quell our rising dis-ease.

Let's now look more closely at contemporary America's views on health to see how our societal quest for wellness can have unintended consequences. Understanding what is in the air will help us understand how Frank Carson could find himself in excellent health but worried about Alzheimer's disease and the pulse he hears throbbing in his ears, searching the mirror for new signs of his age, wondering if the mole on his arm might have turned cancerous. And understanding the cultural climate will also help us to see why our continued pursuit of health may not bring us the sense of well-being we seek.

CHAPTER 5

Our Heightened Health Consciousness

THE QUEST FOR HEALTH and physical well-being is a national priority in contemporary America. We cannot go through a day without having our attention drawn to health issues. The signs are everywhere: in every newspaper and on television, in the physical-fitness boom, in our dieting crazes, and in the emergence of entire industries devoted to health-related products and services. Constantly wondering whether what we are doing is healthful or harmful, we spend vast sums of money on medical care and great amounts of time educating ourselves about our bodies and health. Surveys of what Americans think about and talk about place health and illness at the top of the list. A poll of the readers of *Psychology Today* magazine revealed that 42 percent of the respondents thought about their health more often than just about anything else, including their love lives, their work, and their finances.[1] This is in accord with nationwide polls, which show that 46 percent of the respondents identify "good health" as the greatest single source of happiness, placing it ahead of any other alternative, including "great wealth" and "personal satisfaction from accomplishments." (Women, the elderly, single people, and homeowners are the people who put the greatest premium on good health.)[2]

The personal quest for health seems most intense among people in the middle and upper-middle classes, but it is by no means restricted to them.[3] A 1985 Gallup survey asked a random sample of over 1,000 adults which "healthy changes" they had made in their lives in the past few years.[4] Sixty percent of them said they had adopted a healthier diet, 46 percent had lost weight, 45 percent exercised more, 44 percent said they had learned to control stress on the job, 39 percent reported drinking less alcohol, and 15 percent said they had decreased their cigarette smoking. Overall, 87 percent of the respondents said they had made at least one of these six changes.

Medical images and references to health lace our conversation, the daily news, and our advertisements. Medical stories are "media events." We have only to think, for example, of the frequent heartbreaking appeals for donor organs. When little Amie Garrison, five, of Clarksville, Indiana, required a liver transplant to survive, T-shirts saying HELP US HELP AMIE LIVE were printed up; a country-and-western band helped to raise money; both Indiana senators assisted in trying to locate a donor.[5] And when a donor heart was found for Baby Jesse, a California infant, his parents were given the good news live on nationwide television: "We are donating a heart to the baby," triumphantly announced a spokeswoman for a hospital in Grand Rapids, Michigan. The cameras zoomed in on Baby Jesse's parents as they burst into tears while the audience cheered.[6]

News coverage of each battle in the war on disease is relayed directly from the front lines to an audience anxiously awaiting word of new victories, eager to learn about the newest weapons in our therapeutic armamentarium. The public seems transfixed by the torrent of publicity accompanying every new medical advance, no matter how equivocal the research finding, no matter how experimental the treatment. In a typical instance, when researchers at the National Cancer Institute published a preliminary report on a highly experimental new form of cancer treatment (adoptive immunotherapy), it dominated all three networks' nightly news broadcasts that evening and appeared on the front pages of the nation's newspapers the next morning. The National Cancer Institute's telephone hot line received over 1,000 calls that day. One reason this work was published in such preliminary form in a medical journal was that partial information had already reached the broadcast and print media, through a *Fortune* cover story headlined CANCER BREAKTHROUGH.[7] Researchers are pushed to provide earlier and earlier release of preliminary results, and many now feel free to speculate for public consumption before tentative findings can be critically evaluated or appropriate caveats issued. There is a great sense of urgency about all this, as if we should "interrupt our regularly scheduled programming" with the latest dispatch, experimental data rushed to the broadcasting studio from the laboratory where they were discovered only moments ago, instantaneously translated into life-saving "breakthroughs."

The crusade for health leads us to scrutinize every aspect of daily life for its health implications and consequences: what we eat, how we sleep, where we live, what kind of work we do. The pursuit of the "healthy lifestyle" has become such a prominent avocation that health spas and "fitness resorts" are increasingly popular vacation destinations. About 5 million people went to a spa last year, up twelve-fold from five years ago.[8] Here guests devote every waking moment to the care of the body. There are daily aerobic dance classes; exercise sessions on trampolines, in swimming pools, and in weight rooms; sauna, whirlpool, and massage; nutrition and general health education classes (how to breathe, how to conquer low-back pain, how to reduce stress); and beauty treatments. The menus, in keeping with the emphasis upon health at all costs, list the calories rather than the prices.

Frank Carson found that his entire life was touched by the highly health-conscious culture. This cultural mandate can be a potent amplifier of bodily symptoms; as we have seen, a heightened focus of attention on your body and your health can lead you to feel more ill. In this chapter we will examine

America's heightened health consciousness in this light. But first, in order to see just how and to what extent our society has heightened our awareness of health and made it such a focus of collective attention, we need a historical perspective.

Integrating the Sick into the Social Mainstream

The increasing attention we pay to health and disease arises out of a long historical progression in which sick people have been integrated more and more into the mainstream of society. We now confront the emotionally disturbed, the disfigured and disabled, and the seriously ill more often and at closer range than we did in the past. Increasingly, we see motorized wheelchairs in the street, and we watch disabled people compete in widely publicized sports events. Special needs students join the mainstream in regular classrooms, we deinstitutionalize chronic psychiatric patients so that they can live in their communities, and through the hospice movement, people die outside the hospital, at home. Neighbors receive cancer chemotherapy or kidney dialysis in their own homes. This greater visibility and prominence have been a consciousness-raising experience for people who are not ill or disabled—for the general public at large.

In primitive cultures, the sick person was ostracized and abandoned, even by his own family. He was regarded as the victim of evil forces, such as witchcraft, spirits, or the wrath of a diety. Those who were well believed the sick person posed a threat to their own health, so they fled from him and isolated him in his helplessness and pain.[9]

Later, the Greeks held a different view of sickness, viewing the sick person as inferior and unworthy. Health was regarded as life's greatest gift, its highest blessing, the individual's most important attribute. The ideal man was a harmonious balance of both mental and physical health. Disease, then, was a great misfortune because it removed man from this condition of perfection and balance. The invalid, the cripple, the infirm were inferior. If they regained their health, they became fully worthwhile people again and could reenter society. If recovery was not possible, however, the Greeks saw no sense in medical treatment, and suicide was thought justifiable at that point.[10]

With the coming of Christianity, the sick person took a giant step toward the center of society. Christianity is a religion of saving grace that offers healing and redemption to the sick and the crippled. Whereas the ancients isolated the sufferer, the sick person was integrated into Christian society. Disease came to mean purification, rather than sin or inferiority. Suffering became a means of cleansing the soul; pain fulfilled man by refining his spiritual strength. The sick person now had a privileged status, for he was in a state of grace. Disease was a cross the sufferer carried, for which he would be rewarded after death.[11]

It was in this spirit that the churches began taking up voluntary collections for the sick. After the fourth century, hospitals were built as an expression of Christian charity, and the care of the sick was placed in the hands of religious orders. From the sixth century on, monasteries provided care for the sick as one of their central functions. And beginning in the thirteenth century, Holy Ghost hospitals were built all over Europe.

With the rise of towns and cities, and the growing importance of political citizenship, civil hospitals were started, and the care of the sick fell under the aegis of the state. Medical care increasingly became the responsibility of the community at large. The sick were cared for out of social responsibility rather than religious charity. This movement grew as secular government evolved toward the modern social welfare state.[12]

What about the modern era? From this historical perspective, the most striking thing about the sick person's place in contemporary society is its centrality and its prominence.

We have furthered the historical trend of integrating the sick into the mainstream of society. And we have done more than merely tolerate the sick person; we have enfranchised him. Sickness is now a dispensation entitling the victim to special benefits and privileges. Monetary compensation is provided to the chronically ill and the disabled, as well as preference in qualifying for many kinds of public assistance. We provide workman's compensation, disability insurance, and litigation awards for injury and suffering. We have validated and affirmed the state of being sick, thereby making it more acceptable and more important.

Indeed, disability in the workforce is a veritable epidemic. In 1985, 12 percent of all employable people between the ages of sixteen and sixty-four had received compensation for disability *of at least six months' duration.* The total amount of all payments to the disabled, which includes disability insurance, indemnity programs, and income support, came to $67.4 billion in 1982. The costs of medical care for the disabled added another $51.9 billion on top of this.[13] In the U.S. Postal Service, disability payments for back pain alone consume 0.8 cent out of every 22-cent stamp sold.[14] The medical-disability claims under Social Security Disability Insurance have skyrocketed, more than doubling between 1966 and 1978.[15] Increases in the number of beneficiaries and in the total payments on disability claims have far outpaced the increases in the number of retirees and the amount of money paid to them.[16] In 1970 these disability payments totaled $25 billion. By 1980 they had climbed to $65 billion. And in 1985, just five years later, total disability payments under the Social Security programs approached $100 billion, which amounted to 6 percent of all the personal income earned by nondisabled workers.

This kind of assistance may at times have an unintended and paradoxical consequence: in helping the disabled, we may at the same time perpetuate their impairment. Thus it has been found that the greater the disability benefits offered, the more beneficiaries there will be. As the level of benefits climbs above an individual's expected earnings, then he has a greater and greater incentive to obtain disability coverage, and there is a decreasing likelihood that he will leave the disability rolls.[17] Actuarial data show that people do indeed react differently to the same illness or injury depending upon their disability-insurance coverage. One study, for example, compared policyholders whose coverage was limited to two years of disability benefits following an injury to policyholders whose coverage extended to age sixty-five. The study showed that one-quarter of those who recovered under the former plan would have continued to claim disability benefits had they been insured under the long-term-benefit plan.[18]

We have also made the sick person more visible and more acceptable by substituting illness criteria for means criteria in distributing the benefits of social programs. There has been a trend toward reducing governmental welfare and poverty programs and increasing the assistance to the sick and disabled; being sick or impaired will bring you public assistance, but being poor won't. Nursing homes and custodial-care facilities have replaced almshouses, and the prerequisite for payment of nursing home costs by Medicare is a medical diagnosis. Health rather than wealth also determines whether we qualify for other forms of governmental assistance, such as public housing.[19] A diabetic unable to afford a telephone, for instance, may be given the means to obtain one if his doctor certifies it is necessary for medical management, or he may be allowed to jump to the top of the waiting list for public housing. Likewise, the homeless who are mentally ill have a better chance of finding housing than the homeless who are not.

From his original position of permanent ostracism, the sick person was able to reenter Greek society if he recovered. In the Middle Ages sickness acquired a redeeming value, and the sick person had a privileged status within the Christian community. Subsequently, the public at large assumed responsibility for the care of the sick, and in our time we have steadily given them a more prominent and more advantaged position in the mainstream of society. The result has been to increase the visibility of the sick, to make sickness a more acceptable state, and to heighten the general public's health consciousness. In short, we pay more attention to sick people, and we are more aware of sickness as a state.

Sickness as a Public Event and a Source of Celebrity

As illness has become less stigmatized, personal health has acquired a public quality. Health and illness are no longer confidential or private matters, closely kept family secrets. On the contrary: nowadays you discuss your illnesses with friends over the dinner table; you publicly proclaim your condition, joining with others who are similarly afflicted in mutual support groups; you may even volunteer for a charity crusading to raise money and heighten public awareness of the disorder. Your illness may become one of your most interesting attributes, an important part of your identity, even a way of calling attention to yourself. People are as likely to break the ice at a cocktail party with a gambit about their pulse rate as about their astrological sign, and sickness can even be a means to personal prominence and celebrity.

If you are already a prominent person, your illness may heighten your fame and become a source of publicity. The most intimate details of your anatomy are diagrammed in full color in *Time* and *Newsweek*. When the actor Rock Hudson died so tragically of AIDS, his illness generated more public attention than his acting career had. When Lyndon Johnson called photographers into his room at the Bethesda Naval Hospital in 1965 and proudly pulled up his pajama top to display the scar from his recent gall-bladder surgery, he prefigured this movement toward illness as a public event. In subsequent years we were to receive far more explicit information about Hubert Humphrey's bladder, Betty Ford's breast and her substance abuse problems, and Ronald Reagan's colon and prostate.

Some people have become celebrities solely on the basis of a rare or grotesque disease they have contracted, or achieve renown by undergoing a heroic new therapy such as living for years in a germ-free isolation room. Barney Clark, Baby Fae (the recipient of a transplanted baboon heart), and William Schroeder became international celebrities because of their heart surgery. We followed their clinical courses and their private lives in intimate detail. Baby Fae's funeral was attended by an overflow crowd and was a national television event. William Schroeder was featured on the nightly network news, talking to President Reagan or beginning to ambulate. That we can recall something as trivial as Mr. Schroeder's call for a can of Coors beer testifies to the extent of his fame.

Ted Slavin also exemplified this phenomenon, for his illness became his most important attribute and the organizing principle of his life.[20] In the mid-1950s, Mr. Slavin developed hepatitis from blood transfusions he had received because he suffered from hemophilia. Over time his body began to manufacture particularly high levels of antibodies to the hepatitis virus. When scientists subsequently developed a diagnostic test for hepatitis, large quantities of this antibody were needed, and Mr. Slavin's blood therefore became very valuable. In the years that followed, he donated a great deal of his blood to further medical research and also marketed it commercially, going on to found a successful company dealing in rare blood factors. His awful illness became much more than a lifelong affliction; it also served as his profession and the vehicle for his humanitarianism.

As we've just seen, illness has become one aspect of self-identity, a public event, and at times even a source of celebrity. This, together with our overview of the historical progression of the sick to a more central position in society, prepares us to examine the increased awareness of health and illness that is so prevalent in contemporary America.

The Fitness Boom:
The Race Will Last as Long as We Run It

The Magnitude of the Fitness Movement

The streets are alive with the sound of pounding sneakers, with the grunts of weight training, the hard-rock music of aerobics classes. People are swimming down pool lanes, cycling along park paths and country roads, running on beaches and back streets. "Getting in shape" and "working out" are sacred themes of contemporary life. Strength, endurance, and fitness have become even closer to godliness than cleanliness. Health clubs are cathedrals built to sanctify the body; weight rooms and tracks have become our temples; athletic paraphernalia are our liturgical articles.

The exercise boom is widespread. While reliable data are difficult to obtain, in large-scale surveys, one-third of Americans report engaging in strenuous exercise at least three times a week.[21] Between 31 and 43 million people are serious joggers,[22] up from about 12 million in 1976.[23] Two hundred thirty-three individuals entered the New York City marathon in 1971; ten years later, there were 25,000 applicants for 16,000 places. Ninety percent of runners report that they do it for reasons of physical fitness, viewing it as "living insurance." "We make new Colts out of old forty-fives," says the athletic director of a New York City YMCA.[24] More than 26 million people say they swim regularly,[25] and an estimated 24 million, mostly women, regularly participate in aerobics classes.[26] The fitness movement is especially striking among college women, who have shown new interest in vigorous and even violent sports such as weight lifting and rugby.

The urge to be fit is an economic goldmine. The sporting goods industry is $12.3 billion strong,[27] and its recent performance has been astonishing: the sales of exercise equipment increased 700 percent in the last decade.[28] While not all joggers wear designer headbands, many buy nylon running suits, polypropylene underwear, a pedometer to log mileage, a special wristband with a zipper pocket for the house keys, and a digital stopwatch with a pulse meter built in to monitor heart rate. Athletic shoes alone are a $2.5 to $4 billion market, and although many wear them around the house rather than on the track, the very ubiquity of the uniform of sweats and jogging shoes shows just how fashionable fitness has become.

The fitness boom also fuels a lucrative market in exercise books, records, and videotapes. *Jane Fonda's Workout Book* has sold 1.25 million copies and was number one on the best-seller list for a year. It spawned a record, an audio tape, and four videos.[29] Dr. Kenneth Cooper's book *Aerobics* and its four sequels have sold 7.5 million copies.

The latest status symbol is the home gym. Increasing numbers of homeowners are investing tens of thousands of dollars to set up "fitness centers" in their own basements, complete with racks of dumbbells, arm-curling machines, and stationary bicycles. Sears, Roebuck, which had one simple rowing machine in its catalogs of the 1920s, now devotes thirty-one pages to fitness devices.[30]

A whole new profession has arisen: the fitness instructor. The affluent hire personal trainers who charge as much as $100 an hour, working with clients in their own homes or in gyms that are open twenty-four hours a day, exhorting them to "do just five more" repetitions. In Hollywood, these trainers have joined agents, managers, and publicists as the key employees of many stars. Actress Jamie Lee Curtis observed that "everyone goes to breakfast, lunch, and dinner with their body staffs. They have practically left their families and jobs to be with their pectorals. Life is timed around the trainers or gym."[31]

The Meaning of Exercise

What seems to be going on here is that fitness and physical conditioning have come to signify something far more fundamental than strong hearts and fully expanded lungs: they symbolize strength of character and personal reform. We use rowing machines and exercise bicycles to build up self-confidence, self-image, and our powers of concentration, as well as our biceps and quadraceps. Because physical conditioning (supposedly) demands total commitment and sacrifice, the endurance of pain ("No pain, no gain"), and dehydration and exhaustion, you are a better person this afternoon for having exercised this morning. Beyond any health benefits, we seem to be saying, fitness is a way to purify the soul and become a nobler person.

Running is perhaps the sport that has been the most extensively promoted on this basis. In the 1960s, when droves of middle-aged, overweight, and sedentary men began running for their lives, converts offered testimonials to their "rebirth" and "salvation" through running.[32] The early pioneers who championed running claimed for it powers of spiritual, moral, and personal reform. Two such spiritual founders of the running movement were George A. Sheehan and James F. Fixx. Fixx was thirty-five when he took up running. With its help, he stopped smoking his customary two packs of cigarettes a day and took off sixty pounds. In 1977 he published *The Complete Book of Running,* which became a number-one best-seller and remains the runner's bible. Sheehan, a New Jersey physician, began running at the age of forty-four and became a sort of prophet. In running he discovered an unlimited potential for "self-betterment"; for him it solved a personal life crisis and then became a source of deep personal meaning.[33]

Given the testimonials of the 1960s, running was widely touted in the 1970s for benefits far beyond its medical value. Whereas initially most joggers were men with heart disease who sought improved cardiovascular conditioning, women and healthy young men now were running too.[34] It was said to produce a keener competitive edge on the job, improve one's sex life, and aid in the discovery of one's fullest spiritual and intellectual potential. Kathy Switzer, head of Avon

Cosmetics' Sports Department, said, "I have seen over-weight, unhappy, insecure women develop a confidence through running that helps them take risks and experience joy in their lives. It is a testimony to what the human body can do."[35] Some even looked to running for immortality and immunity from aging, believing that "the race will continue as long as [they] run it."[36] They voiced the belief that they would never die of a heart attack as long as they were able to run a marathon. Control your body, they said, and you control your fate.

This view of athletic conditioning is easier to understand when we look back at Victorian England, where athletics also became a moral and ethical imperative, and fitness took on a larger cultural meaning.[37] Between 1850 and 1880, athletics became a national mania in England. Many of the sports that we pursue today (like soccer, hockey, golf, tennis, and badminton) first became popular then. Matches between university varsity teams began attracting spectators, records began to be kept, formal track-and-field competitions began. Upper-class Englishmen developed a passion for mountain climbing. And, much as today, athletics became big business. Newspapers and magazines followed sports closely; athletic-clothing manufacturers sprang up.

Underlying this sports mania was the Victorian spirit of self-improvement. This was the age of training and the beginning of calisthenics. Sports were seen as a means of achieving health and forging moral development.[38] The Victorians turned athletics from play into work by investing it with higher purpose and meaning. In forcing oneself to meet extreme physical demands, pitting one's strength and endurance against challenges and obstacles, one gained self-knowledge and self-reliance, built courage and fortitude, and forged one's character. The success of English teams in international sporting events came to be equated with British military prowess. "The battle of Waterloo was won on the playing fields of Eton" was a sentiment heartily endorsed.

In our own era, we are witnessing a similar apotheosis of physical fitness and conditioning. Exercise has come to be seen not just as cardiovascular conditioning but as a way to improve mental health and general performance—even as a route to invincibility, immortality, and control over one's medical destiny.

Our Fascination with Nutrition and Dieting

Nutrition

Our health consciousness is also evident in our preoccupation with nutrition and diet. Ours has been characterized as the "Age of Enlitenment": "lite" bread sticks, "lite" pickles, "lite" ketchup, "lite" pancake syrup. And if the product is not "lite," it is "low": low calorie, low sodium, low cholesterol. Recently we've gone low one better with "no": no preservatives, no caffeine, no nitrates, no sulfites. Fifty-seven percent of adult Americans polled say that they are making a real effort to reduce the salt in their diets; 56 percent report trying hard to avoid too much fat; 49 percent claim they try to cut down on sugar; and 46 percent say they avoid high cholesterol foods.[39] Now more than ever, people truly believe that you are what you eat, so that everything seems to be either an elixir or a poison, and reading ingredient labels is a national pastime. Nutrition is so important that the affluent now retain personal dieticians, at $40 per hour, to help them plan their meals.

Every time we sit down at the table, the question on everyone's mind is, Is it good for you? "Health foods" are now a major segment of the retail food industry. The *Wall Street Journal* observed that "nearly everything that consumers eat today is being promoted as healthful or natural. . . . Marketers are responding to the ever-growing cry from consumers that they want to eat more nutritiously."[40] Thus, Campbell's Soup dubbed its product "health insurance." The label of Chicken of the Sea tuna was redesigned: the old label merely described the product as being packed in water, while the new label proudly proclaims it is packed in pure spring water. A consumer survey revealed that the word *natural* in an advertisement boosts sales more than the words *value, convenience, new, flavor,* or *quality.*[41] Almost one-half of the respondents to a Federal Trade Commission–sponsored survey said they would pay more for a food if it were labeled "natural."

The daily diet of many Americans has indeed changed.[42] We are eating more raw vegetables and salads and whole grains. We have substituted fish for beef and skim milk for whole milk. Egg consumption is down (from 402 per person per year in 1945 to 255 in 1985) and that of chicken is up (from 22 pounds per person per year in 1945 to 58 pounds in 1985).[43] Hard liquor is out and bottled water is in.

While we scrupulously avoid some things, we supplement our diet with others. Forty percent of Americans take at least one vitamin or mineral supplement a day, and 11 percent take five or more such supplements each day.[44] Many believe that if small doses of vitamins are good, then huge doses must be lifesaving (though in fact they can be dangerous), and so an estimated 5 to 10 percent of us take megadoses of one or another vitamin.*[45] And in addition to vitamins, minerals such as zinc, iron, and magnesium are widely consumed.

Recently we have become enthralled with calcium, touted as a preventive of osteoporosis, high blood pressure, and cancer. Practically overnight, calcium has been added to orange juice, Tab, cornflakes. The sales of calcium supplements soared from $18 million in 1980 to $240 million in 1986.[46] The infatuation dates from April 1984, when a National Institutes of Health panel pronounced calcium useful in the management of osteoporosis. Dairy producers and the

* This trend was spurred on by Linus Pauling in 1970 with his book on vitamin C and the common cold. It was followed by use of vitamin B_6 for premenstrual tension and vitamin A for cancer prevention.

makers of calcium supplements immediately sponsored an advertising blitz. It bore fruit: when Tums recast its advertising to emphasize its high calcium content ("Tums is sodium free and rich in calcium"), sales jumped 40 percent.

Extreme food fads have long been viewed as attempts to banish our fears of sickness. The difference now is that many onetime fads are no longer restricted to a few fanatics: beliefs formerly held only by fringe groups are now today's conventional wisdom. It used to be a small minority who proclaimed the value of "organic" and "natural" foods, who decried the use of fertilizers and pesticides, who objected to the use of hormones and antibiotics in meat production, and who alleged that processing depleted the nutritional value of foods. Now, in a nationwide survey, 90 percent of those polled considered pesticides, herbicides, additives, and preservatives to be hazards in our foods.[47] About half of them avoid buying certain foods because of these concerns.

Like fitness, good nutrition signifies far more than mere physiology and metabolism: it is believed to be a solution to a range of unpleasant human experiences and difficulties in living. Typical are the claims made in the book *Eat to Succeed:* "The right nutrition can boost endurance and performance . . . help beat executive stress and pump up productivity and creativity at work . . . slow the aging process . . . promote faster healing when ill, and lessen the toxic effects of anesthesia . . . enhance sexual activity, and much more."[48] One of the most successful recent diet books (five months on the best-seller list and with 350,000 hardcover copies in print) is *Dr. Berger's Immune Power Diet.* In addition to promoting the loss of excess poundage, this diet claims to improve your resistance to infectious disease, to enhance happiness, to heighten sexual interest, and to create a more youthful appearance.[49] We want to believe that diet can effect health miracles, banish loneliness, cure anxiety, and eliminate sexual conflicts.

Many of the diet and nutrition books share an evangelical

fervor not unlike that of the authors who were reborn through running. The formerly profligate and sinful author experiences an epiphany, discovers a dietary regimen that becomes his salvation, and then promotes it as gospel. The diet is the key to a new life, not just to better nutrition, and the dieter is born again.

Weight Loss

The nutrition craze is closely tied to a growing obsession with weight. Approximately 40 million people are consciously fighting the battle of the bulge at any one time. Thirty percent of all American women and 16 percent of men went on diets in 1984.[50] Extreme weight-reducing diets are an epidemic among adolescent girls: 9 percent of high school girls have resorted to *total fasting* at some time during their senior year.[51]

Americans spend more than $10 billion annually on diet pills (so-called girth-control pills), diet books, weight-loss classes, diet meals, and other weight-reducing products.[52] There are meal-replacement products available as powders, wafers, and soups; there are high-fiber products; liquid-protein concoctions; starch blockers; and more. Weight-loss programs are flourishing: 25 million people have attended a Weight Watchers meeting, and membership is growing at 15 percent per year.[53]

Since 1970, women's magazines have contained steadily increasing numbers of diet and weight-loss articles.[54] The best-seller lists generally include at least two diet books, promoting an unending succession of name-brand diets—Atkins, Stillman, Pritikin, Scarsdale, Cambridge—as well as those with a gimmick—the water diet, the liquid-protein diet, the rice diet, the grapefruit diet, and on and on.

The obsession with weight loss can be amusing. Diet doctor James J. Julian was quoted in *Time* magazine as saying, "I've walked into the treatment room to find a woman stark naked on the scale. One took off her tiny diamond earrings.

She even exhaled before she looked at the dial."[55] Many experiment to see if standing on a particular corner of the scale will yield more favorable news. Some hope that the uneven floors of their old homes will provide particular spots where the scale registers a pound or two less. Others avoid weighing themselves after a shower because of the minuscule contribution made by wet hair.[56] But as we shall see later, our growing obsession with diet and weight loss has also had more serious and less amusing consequences.

The Mass Media and Health

Television, radio, books, newspapers, and magazines are filled with advice, discussions, and warnings about health. The sheer volume is awesome, from TV "doctors" and full-length documentaries to medical spots on the radio to newspaper columns on health. The Health and Medicine sections of our bookstores swell with each passing month, and a whole new generation of magazines devoted exclusively to health now beckon from every newsstand. A multitude of worthy causes and advocacy groups, both familiar and arcane, clamor through various media outlets for our attention: leukemia, cystic fibrosis, birth defects, Tourette's syndrome. Commercials remind us that we can't be healthy, attractive, or popular without mouthwashes, eyedrops, foot powder, and laxatives.

Radio and Television

Listening to the radio even briefly, one hears an almost infinite number of variations on the same theme: "Health Talk," "Health Line," "Health Report," "Health News," "Health Watch," "Speaking of Health," "Here's to Your Health," "The Medical Journal," "Medical Minute," "Report on Medicine," and so on and so on. They brief us on the debate over mastectomy for breast cancer, help us shop for dental insurance, and discuss the development of artificial skin for treating burns.

The nightly news is suffused with health issues, providing continuing status reports on an artificial organ recipient or the latest tally of AIDS victims. Beyond the segments explicitly devoted to health, the "Lifestyle Report" examines the health consequences of retirement; "Report on Travel" discusses jet lag; "Your Dollars" guides listeners through the financial ins and outs of prepaid health plans. Every Wednesday, reporters pore over the latest edition of the *New England Journal of Medicine,* preparing to disseminate it to millions on Thursday. A spokesman for the Harvard School of Public Health recounted that he had recently attended a luncheon meeting with TV reporters. Before it ended they all rushed out, saying, "This is Wednesday, *New England Journal* day."

Prime-time television includes numerous medical "specials": serious expositions of various health problems. And there are the prime-time medical series themselves, such as *M*A*S*H, St. Elsewhere,* and *Trapper John, M.D.* During the day, the medical soaps such as *General Hospital* and *Days of Our Lives* take the field. Not surprisingly, if one tallies things, it turns out that a disproportionate number of all the characters on television are medical professionals; they are outnumbered only by criminals and law-enforcement figures.[57] Aside from small talk and general business conversation, health is the largest single topic of conversation on daytime television. Among the daytime serials, sickness and injury are the most important and pervasive type of problem portrayed. One-half of all the characters are involved in a health-related occurrence, and one-half of all their pregnancies result in miscarriage.[58] And, of course, the commercial breaks are packed with remedies for headaches and backaches, constipation and diarrhea, sore throats and stuffy noses. Most recently, physicians and clinics themselves have taken to the airwaves to hawk their services.

Books

Were a foreigner to judge us by touring our bookstores, he might conclude that we were a nation of medical students, our cities giant medical schools without walls. Bookstores have huge departments devoted exclusively to health, with separate sections for specific subjects such as allergies, low blood sugar, longevity, vitamins, and women's health. There are guidebooks for choosing a doctor, manuals on how to interact with him, and dictionaries to explain what he says.[59] In 1984, four of the top ten hardcover nonfiction best-selling books dealt with diet or fitness,[60] whereas in 1965, by contrast, none did.[61]

There is a distinct fascination with the body as an object of study and self-examination. The torrent of titles looking at or in the body includes *Body, The Healthy Body, Human Body, The Body in Question, The Body Book, The Body Almanac, Bodywatching, Body Talk,* and on and on. One especially popular genre is the instruction manual for a particular organ system, which attempts to arm the reader with a complete knowledge of his anatomy and physiology. Examples include *Your Thyroid, The Breast, The Slipped Disc,* and *The Brain.* As *Prevention* magazine reminds us, "Our bodies—the most complex and delicate machines we own—don't come with any operating instructions at all."[62] This corporeal fascination is exemplified by a television message, sponsored by the American Liver Foundation, that aims to incite appreciation and respect, if not downright affection, for our livers. It begins with silence, followed by a grave voice: "The sound you don't hear is your liver, hard at work. . . . It's the most remarkable, uncomplaining organ in your body. . . . It's your liver, performing over 5,000 vital functions every night and every day." The announcement closes with a pitch for a booklet enabling you to "learn how to take care of your liver."

Another popular genre is the personal testimonial, the

prototype being Norman Cousins's *Anatomy of an Illness As Perceived by the Patient,* which was on the *New York Times* best-seller list for forty weeks. Individuals, usually famous, confess their own private struggles with various afflictions, taking readers on a tour of their personal world of suffering and disability.* They offer inspirational images of recovery and hope, though sometimes of despair as well. There is a particular interest in the wounded healer, i.e., in physicians' revelations of their own illnesses, seen in such titles as *A Physician Faces Cancer Himself* and *Stroke, A Doctor's Personal Story of His Recovery.*

Magazines and Newspapers

Several magazines cater to the health market, among them *Prevention,* which was founded in the 1950s and has a world-wide circulation of 2.5 million copies, and the more recent *American Health* and *Fit.* In addition, medical news and advice figure prominently throughout the rest of the popular press; most publications have columnists and correspondents whose beat is medicine. A typical issue of *Readers Digest* (March 1986) contains four feature articles on health: "Ten Great Myths of Personal Fitness," "The Dismal Truth about Teen-Age Health," "Our Toxic-Waste Time Bomb," and "Radioactivity: The New-Found Danger in Cigarettes." The emphasis is on disease prevention and the avoidance of health dangers; the underlying message is that we can actually avoid sickness if we remain alert and well-informed and take all the right precautions.

The point here is that the mass communications media have lately focused more and more on health and disease. In so doing, they direct our attention increasingly to our bodies and to illness, and reflect and reinforce our heightened health consciousness.

---

* Some examples are *Reprieve* by A. Demille (Garden City, NY: Doubleday, 1981); *Heart-Sounds* by M. W. Lear (New York: Simon and Schuster, 1980); *A Coronary Event* by M. Halberstam and S. Lesher (Philadelphia: Lippincott, 1976); and *No Laughing Matter* by J. Heller and S. Vogel (New York: Putnam, 1986).

The Growing Health Economy

Nowhere else do we declare our heightened health consciousness more than in our spending habits. It is no secret that Americans have been spending more and more on health care. In 1970, our total national health expenditures were $75 billion. By 1980, the bill had more than tripled, to $248 billion. And in 1986, only six years later, our expenditures totaled $465 billion.*[63] These figures exceed the total domestic sales of all automobiles (manufactured both abroad and at home) and are greater than the combined sales of our four largest corporations.[65]

The most significant point about the rise in health-care expenditures is that it has been *relative* and not just *absolute:* we are spending proportionately more of our income on health. In 1970, health and medical care made up 7.4 percent of our Gross National Product. By 1980 the figure had increased to 9.1 percent. In 1986, health accounted for 10.8 percent of the GNP.[66] This means that the health-care sector absorbs more than one-twelfth of our nation's total economic production. Put another way, the average American works more than one month a year just to pay for his health care.[67] This explosion in health-care costs is paralleled by an increase in the number of health-related jobs. The health-care industry now employs over 5 million people, so that one out of every fifty of us goes to work each day in a medical or allied-health field.[68]

These figures, moreover, include only health expenditures in the strictest sense, being composed of the costs of personal medical care, biomedical research, the construction of medical facilities, administration, and the like. As such, they constitute only a portion of the overall health-related econ-

---

* We have been buffeted by inflation during much of this period, so these figures were recalculated in constant dollars to take this into account. The same kind of precipitous rise was still evident. The best single measure of health-care expenditures is the per capita outlay in constant dollars. This has gone from $292 in 1970 to $397 in 1980 to $431 in 1986.[64]

omy. There is in addition an enormous arena of nonmedical health care, which at its most malignant includes medical quackery, a giant, well-organized, and sophisticated $10-billion industry.[69] Always prevalent—Pliny prescribed eating a mouse a week to prevent toothaches—medical quackery is growing at an alarming rate.[70] Its resources now include computerized mass mailings, slick television commercials, and phony foundations supplying "scientific" information.

It is important to recognize that rising medical costs have diffused throughout the entire economy. None of us has remained immune because most of the money spent on medical care does not come directly out of the patient's pocket; it comes instead from all of us through our taxes, our health-insurance premiums, and the prices of other goods and services.* Because of health insurance and third-party reimbursement, our own purchases of medical care are subsidized by others. And conversely, even if we never see a doctor or visit an emergency room, we pay part of the bills incurred by our neighbors who do. Health-insurance premiums have become one of the biggest costs of doing business, comprising about half of all the fringe benefits industry pays to its workers. In 1981 General Motors spent $3,270 per employee for health-insurance premiums,[72] paying more per annum to Michigan Blue Cross and Blue Shield than to United States Steel.[73] At the Chrysler Corporation, the cost of health insurance added $600 to the purchase price of each automobile.[74]

Health insurance in itself fuels the demand for more health care, much as we saw when we discussed the way disability insurance benefits perpetuate one's disabled status.

---

* Of the nation's total personal-health-care bill, 42 percent comes from public funds and 26 percent from third-party payers (insurance carriers, private industries, and private philanthropy). Only 32 percent comes directly out of the consumer's pocket. This represents a dramatic change, since in 1966 the patient himself bore 51 percent of medical-care costs.[71]

When a consumer does not pay the total cost of a product or service, he will consume more of it than he would if he paid the whole bill himself. Thus the extension of medical-insurance benefits results in greater utilization of medical care, and another round of cost increases.

This is not to suggest that health-insurance coverage should be diminished or even that our health expenditures should be reduced. It is only to point out that the growth of health insurance and third-party payment heightens health consciousness in two ways: it gives those of us who are not sick an important financial stake in the treatment of those of us who are, and it results in more of us going to the doctor more often.

Health as a Supervalue

Our increased devotion to health is evident in the ways we spend our time and our money, in the orthodoxy of the healthy lifestyle, in the messages issuing from the mass media, and in the prominence of health concerns in daily conversation. Behind this devotion lies the new ideology that health signifies almost everything good and desirable in life. It is summed up in the cheery contemporary adage "When you have your health, you have everything."*

Health is no longer thought of merely as the absence of disease; rather, it is viewed as something positive, a generalized state of physical and mental well-being—of "wellness." We emphasize health so much because for us it means self-actualization, personal fulfillment, and a multitude of other desirable attributes such as self-esteem and self-confidence.[76] We think that good health means enhanced work performance and productivity, optimism and confidence, and greater social attractiveness and sexuality. The healthy, like

* Realizing that other cultures do not value health so highly casts our heightened health consciousness into higher relief: in India, for instance, a greater value is placed on achieving religious purity; the English value living in adherence to the law more highly; in the USSR, the good of the state is more important.[75]

the wealthy, have an elevated status because we take their health to be an outward sign of willpower, of their success in "getting their act together." We think health automatically brings satisfaction with life and optimism about the future, and we feel that in guarding and improving our health we will be satisfying a far wider range of human needs and goals.[77]

Because health has become synonymous with overall well-being, it has become an end in itself, a paramount aim of life. Good health is now the object of conscious, sustained, and deliberate endeavor. Health is no longer valued only because it is a means to other fundamental personal goals, such as professional accomplishment or raising a family. It substitutes for them. The quest for the healthy lifestyle, our pursuit of physical fitness, our dieting, and our growing medical expenditures all embody this view of health as an end in itself. Out of our heightened health consciousness then, health emerges with the status of a "supervalue" or "pan-value,"[78] an overarching priority of life.

Living a meaningful life has thus been reduced to a health problem. Health has become an imperative, like a religious or moral code, which dictates specific norms of conduct. As the astute sociologist Robert Crawford has written, "Healthy behavior has become the paradigm for good living. Healthy men and women become model men and women."[79] We use health norms to judge how people should behave and how life should be lived: how we spend our income, what we read, how we sleep and work and play, and what we eat and drink. As people in the past sought to lead a "religious life," we now seek the healthy lifestyle. Attaining a state of wellness is like attaining a state of grace. In a sense, we've replaced the religious quest for the salvation of our souls with the secular quest for the salvation of our bodies. For many, the highest purpose of human activity is not to purify the soul, but to purify the body. The imperative is not to do good works, but to be good to your body. As Marshall Becker has written, "Health promotion . . . is a new religion, in which we worship ourselves, attribute good health to our devoutness, and view illness as just punishment for those who have not yet seen the way."[80]

We spoke earlier of four factors that amplify feelings of ill health. Attention was one of these. Our culture's heightened health consciousness amplifies private health concerns through this mechanism of attention. Society's increased awareness of health serves to redirect the attention of its citizens to their bodies, their symptoms, and their ailments. And we have already seen how this sort of attention can amplify people's feelings of malaise. In succeeding chapters, we will explore other features of our culture that also serve to amplify individuals' private concerns about illness.

CHAPTER 6

The Medicalization of America

OUR LIFE CIRCUMSTANCES and the situations we are in shape the way we assess our health and how sick we feel, as discussed in chapter 2. The culture is a prism through which our personal health concerns are refracted; it provides the clues we use to determine the meaning and significance of our afflictions. One such cultural clue is a progressive medicalization. We increasingly think of daily life in medical terms, have reclassified many indesirable or painful aspects of life as diseases, and have vastly expanded the role of the patient.

Visiting the Doctor More

"See your doctor early and often" is a dictum we have taken to heart. The average American woman visited a physician 5.7 times in 1983 (i.e., almost once every two months), and the average man went 4.4 times.[1] Eighty percent of us saw a doctor at least once that year. By contrast, in 1930, one-half of all Americans did not visit a physician, and those who went averaged only two and one-half visits.[2]

New groups of people have begun going to doctors in the last one hundred years, people who did not generally consult them before. The dying and the elderly have always received medical attention, but people with lesser complaints, especially women, were generally treated at home.[3] In the modern era, however, younger women began to seek medical care for themselves, and by the 1920s, women visited doctors more frequently than men. As mothers, these young women began bringing in their children as well, so that children were discovered as patients. Earlier, even in the late 1800s, there had been a casualness about infant death because it was so common. Parents readily withdrew their devotion from a young child once he became seriously ill because of the high likelihood that he would die. As infant mortality declined, however, and each child stood a better chance of surviving his early years, parents let themselves become more attached to their infants; and when children became sick, rather than passively awaiting the outcome, mothers now snatched them up and bundled them off to the doctor.[4]

Nowadays, office visits are on the upswing because, as Edward Shorter described in his historical study of the doctor-patient interaction, *Bedside Manners,* we have become more and more willing to take minor symptoms and trivial illnesses (such as colds, sinus complaints, musculoskeletal symptoms, and digestive problems) to doctors.* That is, we are now more likely to consider life's everyday infirmities to be disorders. Shorter estimates that women with urinary-tract complaints are five times more likely to seek medical attention now than they were in the 1920s.[6] Upper-respiratory-tract infections are now the most common single disease encountered in general medical practice, and most patients with such infections see their doctors within *one week* of the onset of their colds; 3 to 6 percent of them even go within the *first day* of developing symptoms.[7] This is true even though it is well known that if treated vigorously by a physician the common cold will disappear within seven days, whereas if left alone it will subside over the course of a week.

---

* Shorter noted a similar phenomenon in England, where between 1847 and 1947, as the health status of the population increased, the proportion of patients coming to the doctor with minor complaints increased.[5]

In 30 to 60 percent of all visits made to primary-care physicians and general practitioners today, no serious medical cause can be found to account for the patient's symptoms. And if we focus not on the visits but on the patients, we find that 25 to 40 percent of those who are being cared for in general medical outpatient settings have no serious medical diseases whatsoever. Thus we have a panoply of people who are patients because they are troubled by symptoms, but who are not seriously sick. Some are the "worried well" whom we discussed in chapter 3. But we see them in doctors' waiting rooms, in line to have X rays taken, at the drugstore picking up prescription medication.

Preventive Medicine: Medical Care for the Healthy

We have expanded patienthood in another way. With the advent of preventive medicine, we go to doctors when we feel healthy. We go for routine checkups, for health education, for genetic screening and counseling, and for health-hazard appraisals.

The concept of detecting disease before it manifests itself is at the heart of preventive medicine. Thus people who feel well go to doctors for diagnostic procedures, such as mammograms, which can disclose hidden disorders. Every corner of the body can be probed, every organ visualized, with these new diagnostic techniques. Nuclear Magnetic Resonance Imaging (NMR), for example, reveals the moment-to-moment metabolic changes that occur almost anywhere in the body; with it we can practically visualize the chemistry of a single thought. Diagnostic ultrasound reveals the heart valves opening and closing with each heartbeat and egg cells ripening in the ovary, and with it we can spy on the unborn fetus as he yawns. Sophisticated genetic screening and chromosome analyses allow us to predict for potential parents the odds that their offspring will have certain hereditary diseases. Because these procedures are safe, painless, and noninvasive, they are employed extensively, even when there is little likelihood of discovering disease.

These innovations in diagnostic technology permit us to probe beneath ostensible good health to detect hidden pathology of which the individual is unaware. This newfound capability erodes our confidence in the state of apparent good health, because outward appearances may be deceiving: we may actually be sick and simply not know it. The result is that we can no longer trust the intuitive and subjective sense of well-being and good health as much as we once could.

Seeming good health has also been medicalized as a result of our knowledge of risk factors that predispose healthy people to developing various diseases in the future. Knowing an individual's personal habits, the medical problems that run in his family, and the results of some laboratory tests, we can calculate his chances of developing various common diseases. It is then possible to counsel him in lowering these risk factors, helping him to do things today that will lessen his chances of getting sick tomorrow. Thus we now obtain medical care not only to determine what is wrong with us (diagnosis), but also to determine what may go wrong in the future (a health-risk or health-hazard appraisal). We have redefined the notion of "patient" to include not just the sick person, but the potentially sick person as well, and we have expanded the purview of medical care from existing disease to future disease.

With this new concern about diseases to which we may someday fall prey, even though we are healthy at present, personal habits that were devoid of medical implications in the past, and daily activities that we once took for granted, are now thought of in terms of their future health consequences. Such awareness carries with it an obligation to alter the pathogenic behavior. Preventive medicine aimed at heart disease is a good example. The steak dinner we used to enjoy while oblivious to any possible health implications now seems a form of medical suicide, as if we were overdosing on cholesterol and fueling a time bomb planted in our chests.

We do not wish to imply, of course, that there are no health benefits from all this. Quite to the contrary, preventive medicine has been a major factor in improving our health status. But the psychological effect is the same as that resulting from our expanded diagnostic capability: feeling healthy is no longer an adequate justification for putting concerns about illness out of mind. The purview of medical care has widened to include milder ailments, hidden or occult disease, and future disorders. A far-reaching medicalization results as more and more of life is infused with health implications. We think of ourselves as patients even when we feel well.

Making Differences into Diseases

We have also expanded the boundaries of what we consider to be diseases. Accordingly, as Leon Kass writes in *The Public Interest,* "All kinds of problems now roll into the doctor's door, from sagging anatomies to [potential] suicides, from unwanted childlessness to unwanted pregnancy, from marital difficulties to learning difficulties, from genetic counseling to drug addiction, from laziness to crime."[8] What is usual is increasingly regarded as healthy, and differences between people are more and more often defined in terms of disease. We now consult doctors with problems that we did not used to think of as medical disorders: deviant behavior such as alcoholism, drug addiction, and impulsive violence; undesirable bodily characteristics such as baldness, small breasts, and aging skin; and maladaptive personality traits.

Observers such as Eliot Freidson, Thomas Szasz, and Ivan Illich consider such medicalization a harmful usurpation by organized medicine of the management of suffering and distress that should be met by personal, social, and community responses. Medical professionals, they suggest, have encouraged an inappropriate dependence upon the medical-care system, which has eroded the community resources and institutions that would better serve people taking care of each other. Medicalization, they argue, is professional self-aggrandizement, the expansion of professional dominance and authority over people's lives. But in this book, medicalization is viewed more as a result of two other factors: the rising demands of a populace increasingly obsessed with health and disease, and biomedical advances themselves.

It is important to appreciate the role of biomedical advances in fueling this process of medicalization: we are now able to alter human biology and behavior and mental activity in ways only dreamed of a few short years ago. Many troubling conditions have been medicalized, then, because we have acquired the capability to "treat" them.

The Medicalization of Maladaptive Behavior

There has been a historic trend toward viewing socially unacceptable behavior such as alcoholism, drug addiction, and interpersonal violence as medical disorders. In the distant past, such maladaptive behavior was regarded as sinful. Repentance and expiation were therefore prescribed. Later, this behavior was considered criminal, and punishment became the remedy. Most recently, we have come to view it as a disorder requiring medical treatment.[9] Much maladaptive and deviant behavior is now thought to have specific biological causes over which free will and religious devotion have little influence. One may think of the law as dealing with deviant acts for which we are held accountable, and medicine as dealing with deviant acts for which we are not held responsible.[10] As a result, some argue, in the second half of the twentieth century, medicine has come to rival religion and law as the major institutions of social control.[11]

ALCOHOLISM

We have long known of the dire medical consequences of excessive alcohol intake, and we have always considered it appropriate for doctors to treat the alcoholic's liver cirrhosis and his infections. But what about the *person* who drinks too much, who gets drunk and then behaves unacceptably? If he gets into fights while intoxicated, or tells off his boss, is this a voluntary loss of control for which he is responsible, or is his behavior a symptom of a disease, the inevitable result of alcohol's effect upon the brain? In short, does the deviant behavior result from the drink or the drinker?[12]

In the nineteenth century, drunkenness was viewed as moral depravity. This view contributed to the rise of the temperance movement, and in 1919 we enacted Prohibition. But Prohibition was repealed in 1933, and the disease model of alcoholism—that is, alcoholism as a psychiatric disorder—grew in prominence.[13] It has been suggested that the rise of the disease model came from the need for a new form of social control of drinking once it was no longer a crime, since it remained socially undesirable. In the decades that followed, several developments fostered the acceptance of the idea that drinking behavior was itself a disease, including scientific research and the growth of Alcoholics Anonymous.

In the late 1960s and early 1970s there was widespread decriminalization of public drunkenness, and with it came legislative mandates for treatment rather than punishment. This resulted in an enormous increase in the numbers of alcoholics taken to general-hospital emergency rooms and admitted to state mental hospitals, since there were no longer "drunk tanks" in which to detain them.[14]

NARCOTIC ADDICTION

Narcotic, or opiate, addiction has had a similar history. In the nineteenth century, drug addiction was considered immoral and evil, a weakening of the will. But in the early twentieth century, drug addiction became a much more prevalent problem.[15] The government tried to control opium use by regulating its sale and by designating its use for non-therapeutic purposes as criminal and illegal. But criminalizing it did not stem the rising tide. Quite the contrary, an addict subculture emerged and a criminal drug underworld came into being. Addicts began filling the prisons. Criticism of the criminal approach to the problem grew, and in the mid-1950s calls increased for medical alternatives. At this point methadone was discovered and hailed as the medical solution to the problem. It was embraced by policymakers, and we saw the rapid growth of methadone programs and inpatient and outpatient drug-treatment centers directed by physicians. The control of addicts had shifted from the law-enforcement system to the medical-care system, and the emphasis shifted from punishment to treatment.[16] Opiate use has remained illegal, however, so at present addiction is considered to be both criminal and pathological.

VIOLENCE

Increasing numbers of violent individuals have been committed to mental hospitals rather than incarcerated in prisons, the rationale being that we rehabilitate individuals rather than simply punish them. The responsibility for these persons has thus been shifted from the criminal-justice system to the mental-health system. The insanity defense is invoked more frequently, and defendants more often plead incompetence to stand trial on psychiatric grounds.[17] More recently, there has been a countermovement back toward stricter and more punitive responses to violent behavior, with the reinstitution of the death penalty and mandatory sentencing, but medicalization still persists alongside this countermovement.

Criminals with a history of impulsive violence, and people unable to control their aggressive and hostile urges have been studied psychiatrically and neurologically. Some have subtle brain disorders that might play a role in their violent behavior. Temporal-lobe epilepsy, for example, sometimes results in long-term personality changes, which include unpremeditated violent outbursts. Similarly, post-traumatic stress syndrome has been invoked as a cause of interpersonal violence in some Viet Nam veterans. In other cases, the medical grounds are more shaky: violent criminals in rising numbers claim that their acts resulted from toxins to which they were exposed. In a particularly celebrated example, Dan White pleaded "diminished capacity" in connection with the shooting death of the mayor of San Francisco in 1978. Mr. White's lawyers contended that a diet of sugary junk food aggravated underlying psychological problems, an argument referred to as the "Twinkie defense."

CHILD ABUSE

Child abuse has occurred throughout history, but only in the last twenty-five years has it been clearly defined as a medical problem.[18] In the past, when physicians treated injuries inflicted on children by their parents, they did not inquire into the cause or recognize the abuse for what it was. Then, in medical journals of the 1950s, certain characteristic patterns of physical trauma in children came to be recognized as resulting from assaults made upon them. When reports of this filtered into the mass media, concern for abused children began to increase, and in the early 1960s the term *battered child* entered our lexicon. Physicians now had a diagnostic label for a specific condition and began to recognize the condition as such in their patients.

The newly recognized child abuser was thought of as having a psychological disorder, at first based upon the simple notion that "anybody who would do a thing like that must be sick." Subsequent evidence of abusers' psychopathology and abnormal upbringing brought additional support for this view, and we endorsed treatment rather than punishment for them. Child abuse was understood to be a social and psychiatric problem, the battered-child syndrome became a medical diagnosis, and the abuser joined the swelling ranks of patients in our society.[19]

CHILDHOOD HYPERACTIVITY

Poor performance in school is an example of maladaptive behavior that was traditionally thought of as only undesirable but has now been medicalized as well. In many instances, a student's poor academic or social performance is the result of a problem in cognitive development or of a psychiatric disorder, and such a child is now more likely to be diagnosed as hyperactive or as having a learning disability or a conduct disorder. In the past, the same child's behavior would have been attributed to laziness, rebelliousness, or even stupidity.

Childhood hyperactivity (also called minimal brain dysfunction) in particular has only become a psychiatric diagnosis in the last twenty-five years, but it is now the most commonly diagnosed behavioral problem of childhood. Before, children who exhibited the symptoms (inattention and distractibility, difficulty concentrating on and finishing tasks, impulsivity, and excessive physical activity) were called disruptive, disobedient, or antisocial.[20] The accepted response to their deviant behavior was disciplinary and was administered by teachers and school authorities and by parents. Now such children are more likely to be diagnosed as hyperactive and treated by doctors with medication (often with a striking improvement in their behavior).

But in this case, as in some of the others we've discussed, we may have gone overboard in our zeal to invoke a medical explanation for troublesome behavior. As many as 10 to 15 percent of children are now being diagnosed as hyperactive, and at times this has been little more than a medical name for behavior that is maladaptive and objectionable.[21] Similarly, the chief of psychiatry at a medical school, to whom failing medical students are frequently referred for evaluation, observed: "So often they are sent to me by the dean or a department chairman who suspects that they are depressed or using drugs; but in my experience, the problem often turns out to be simply that they are just not motivated enough or aren't capable of doing the work. "

How has this come about? With the rise of scientific medicine, doctors increasingly became a major source of information about child rearing. And when viewed through medically trained eyes, intellectual and behavioral traits that may not be pathological but instead represent developmental delays, or are within the range of normal, or result from turmoil within the family tend to be seen as disorders.[22] Increasingly now, we recognize that differences among children can reflect individual variability more than disease, but our general inclination to apply medical diagnoses to deviant behavior still stands as evidence of our society's sweeping medicalization.

The Medicalization of Physical Appearance and Bodily Functioning

UNATTRACTIVENESS

Physical characteristics that used to be considered simply unattractive or undesirable have become medically and surgically alterable, and so unappealing features are now regarded as if they were disfiguring deformities. Such people are not "sick" in the traditional sense, but medical care is employed to enhance their looks or create an impression of youthfulness. Cosmetic surgeons transplant hair to "treat" baldness, implant silicone to enlarge breats or produce a more Grecian nose, tighten baggy stomachs, and siphon off body fat.

Plastic surgery is one of the fastest-growing medical specialties. It is estimated that there were 500,000 cosmetic operations performed in the United States in 1986, up from 300,000 in 1981.[23] The most popular of these are liposuction (the removal of fat from beneath the skin by suction) and breast augmentation, which was performed on 95,000 women in 1984 (thus expanding our nation's feminine pulchritude by 13,000 gallons of silicone gel).[24] But women are not the only customers: the proportion of men undergoing cosmetic surgery has risen from 5 to 20 percent over the last ten years.[25] And their operations are no longer limited to hair transplants, as they once were. Nor are these men only in white-collar occupations; firemen, truck drivers, and factory workers are having their noses recontoured, the bags removed from under their eyes, and the fat vacuumed from beneath their chins. Even orthodontic treatment is now used more to treat people's appearance than to cure diseases of the jaw: 80 percent of those who go to orthodontists do so for cosmetic reasons.[26]

OBESITY

We have medicalized obesity by reducing it to a disease. To be sure, obesity does pose a medical danger: obese people are more likely to die from heart disease, some cancers, and diabetes, and they are at greater risk for high blood pressure. But being overweight, in and of itself, was never before considered a disease.

Our contemporary culture has increasingly found obesity unattractive, but historically, female plumpness has generally been esteemed, viewed as a sign of prosperity and wealth, of fertility and strength. Only when food is plentiful do dieting and slimness come into vogue. The difference between our current ideal of thinness and the ideal of the past is illustrated by the contrast between the svelte and elongated women of Modigliani and the ripe and ample nudes of Peter Paul Rubens.

While being slender has been desirable for much of this century, this preference has intensified in the last fifteen years or so.[27] Madame Tussaud's wax museum in London asks its visitors which woman among those represented they think has the most beautiful figure. In 1970 they picked Elizabeth Taylor, but by 1976, Twiggy was selected. A glance at the contemporary standards of feminine beauty displayed in the movies and in fashion magazines confirms that extreme thinness is "in." Even the *Playboy* magazine centerfold models have become progressively thinner since the magazine began publishing in 1953, as have the Miss America contestants.[28]

An aesthetic imperative toward thinness fostered our viewing obesity as undesirable, but it was the recognition of obesity as a health risk factor and the evolution of medical treatments (such as gastrointestinal bypass surgery and the surgical removal of fat) that caused us to reclassify this so-called undesirable physical characteristic as a disease.

OLD AGE

Geriatric medicine is a new and valuable medical specialty concerned with the medical disorders of the elderly. But we have gone beyond this to medicalize old age in another way, by creating a popular myth that the aging process itself is some sort of disorder that is susceptible to medical treatment. This myth had its origins in genuine advances made in the study of the elderly. These revealed that some of the complaints prevalent among old people were actually due to disorders that had previously gone unrecognized and untreated and were not simply manifestations of the aging process itself, as had been assumed. But the discovery that some of the symptoms of older people stem from treatable disorders has been popularized, promoted, and publicized in ways that transform aging itself from a vexation into a disorder, "a medical problem that your doctor can do something about." As in the case of obesity, the reclassification of old age as a disorder has been fueled by a growing dislike of certain bodily characteristics of aging. (Our unease about aging will be discussed in more detail in chapter 8.)

LIFE'S MALADIES

Uncomfortable everyday physical experiences are being redefined as pathological. In other words, the wear and tear of daily life is increasingly viewed as sickness. Benign, though troublesome, dysfunctions such as fatigue, drowsiness, occasional impotence, forgetfulness, jet lag, and motion sickness are increasingly thought of as disorders and treated medically.

We may have had the symptom for a long time but viewed it as an inherent part of living, one of life's inevitable discomforts. We hadn't thought of ourselves as sick until influenced by a massive publicity blitz about some newly identified but still vague condition, which suggests that the symptom is pathological. There are a number of such conditions around about which we have very little scientific knowledge, for example, "yeast infections," "ecological allergies," "chronic mononucleosis," and "hypoglycemia." They are often quasi-diseases, part real, part fiction. While they may truly afflict a small number of people, they are heartily embraced by a great many more who are seeking to attribute their discomfort to disease, hoping to find thereby that whatever troubles them is treatable. These people are indeed suffering, but in the past their suffering was not thought of as a medical disease.

Fatigue is a good example. While fatigue can be pathological—that is, a symptom of illness—far more often it is a perfectly normal part of life. But we now tend to think of being weary and tired as an abnormal and treatable symptom. For example, a new book, *Women and Fatigue,* promises "effective solutions to this very real problem."[29] In advertisements the author says, "I wrote this book . . . as one who has personally struggled with chronic fatigue—and won. The causes of fatigue can be found and every woman can learn how to conquer them."

Chronic mononucleosis (chronic Epstein-Barr virus infection, or CEBV syndrome) illustrates this confusion between a normal dysfunction and a disease symptom. This condition, only recently identified, is characterized by chronic and profound fatigue, but its nature remains unclear and its very existence is not entirely established. We don't know how significant or widespread it is, we don't know how to distinguish it from simple tiredness, nor do we know how reliable or valid the diagnostic tests for it are. Yet chronic mononucleosis has immediately been elevated to the status of a major public-health problem. Large numbers of tired people relabel their complaint as pathological fatigue and consult doctors after having already diagnosed themselves as suffering from chronic mononucleosis. They have formed dozens of self-help support groups. One such group, whose leader describes her own condition as "a living hell," reports that it gets 1,000 letters a day and has 12,000 members.[30] This massive groundswell indicates just how rapidly some people can seize upon a new diagnostic label to explain a longstanding discomfort. In part we do this because it means that an intransigent and troublesome problem might now be cured.

Premenstrual syndrome (PMS) is similar: a medical disorder undoubtedly exists, but the dividing line between it and normal menstrual discomfort is unclear. The wish to see our disturbing sensations as symptoms of disease is evident in public proclamations such as this portion of an advertisement: "In the last few years, research has revealed that much of your tension, irritability, and discomfort can be symptoms of PMS."[31] As a result, PMS tends to be overdiagnosed, and some women whose menstrual periods are distressing but not abnormal now believe that they are sick with a disease. Many of the women attending PMS clinics report symptoms that are indistinguishable from those of women who do not consult physicians because they do not consider themselves to be sick. In part this medicalization of menstruation stems from our hope that medical science will be able to ameliorate its most distressing phenomena. But while some of these symptoms may eventually be treatable, we did not used to think of them as such, and reclassifying them as abnormal, transforming premenstrual "blues" into premenstrual "syndrome," influences how we think about health, disease, and our bodies.

Other disorders, more clearly mythical, are created by public-relations campaigns, advertising, the media, and physicians and hucksters who pander to the public clamor for medical breakthroughs. Disorders such as hypoglycemia, yeast infections, and ecological illness exist more in the public consciousness and in common parlance than in clinical reality. For example, hypoglycemia, or "low blood sugar," with rare exceptions, is not a significant medical disorder. Many healthy people experience transient lightheadedness, tremulousness, sleepiness, and difficulty thinking following meals. But not infrequently, these normal phenomena are incorrectly judged to be pathological and therefore mislabeled as hypoglycemia.[32]

Some of life's miseries and nuisances have actually yielded to medical advance. Conditions such as insomnia, stuttering, and unsatisfactory sexual performance may be included here. We have always had trouble sleeping, but only recently has a whole group of "sleep disorders" entered the medical lexicon, along with new treatments for them. Insomnia used to be a condition we simply endured, or for which we tried a favorite folk remedy, had an extra highball, or used a non-specific sedative. Now, however, we can diagnose different types of insomnia by monitoring the brain's electrical activity in a sleep laboratory. A common malady that did not garner much clinical attention is now the subject of extensive medical evaluation and treatment. Something similar has happened with sexual performance. Sexual dissatisfaction has become sexual "dysfunction," as it has become possible to help people with problems as major as impotence and frigidity and as minor as the inability to have simultaneous orgasms.

NORMAL BODILY PROCESSES

The ultimate extension of this trend has been reached with the development of medical techniques to "treat" perfectly normal characteristics in some desired way. One such technique is gender-altering surgery. Transsexuals, individuals who have a lifelong, unshakable conviction that they are actually members of the opposite sex, can have their secondary sexual characteristics suppressed with hormones and be transformed surgically from anatomically normal males into females, or vice versa. Medical techniques have also been employed to enhance the body's normal physiological capacities: anabolic steroids improve the football player's strength; autologous blood transfusions ("blood doping") give the marathoner greater endurance; stimulant drugs can suspend the body's normal requirements for food and rest. Nowhere is medicine's newly acquired power to intervene in normal biology more awesome than in the area of reproductive function. Tubal ligation and vasectomy block the normal process of conception, and bring people who are not sick in any sense into the doctor's office. Medication and techniques such as in vitro fertilization permit couples formerly considered to be simply and irrevocably childless to be counseled and treated for a disorder, "infertility." And in vitro fertilization has the potential of allowing couples to choose the sex, or even the physical characteristics, of their child, thereby interjecting medicine even further into the normal birth process.

The Medicalization of Emotional Distress

We have also widened the range of psychological suffering subject to medical treatment. After the Boston Red Sox lost the 1986 World Series, the social-work department of a Boston hospital offered a self-help group for depressed employees; more than 150 people showed up to talk about their feelings.[33] Psychotherapy is advised for children anxious about the arrival of a new sibling, for families whose houses have been burglarized, for people "suffering" from baldness. A perusal of the *Boston Globe* classified advertisements on any given day reveals medical and psychological support groups for head-injury patients, stroke patients, herpes patients, and sickle-cell anemia patients; for the families of people suffering from dementia and schizophrenia; for the divorced, separated, bereaved; for pregnant women, new mothers, mothers of toddlers, and single mothers; and for the victims of assault or incest.[34] Such groups may be extremely helpful; it is only that thinking of these misfortunes and difficulties as medically treatable represents a shift in our outlook on life's tribulations. In the past, these miseries were burdens, tragedies, curses, or another of life's bitter pills to be sure, but they did not transform the afflicted into candidates for psychiatric therapy.

While most patients who come to psychiatrists or other mental-health professionals are troubled by true psychiatric disorders and serious mental suffering, some now receive treatment for personal characteristics or difficulties in living that in the past we did not think were medically treatable. Salesmen request treatment for their fears of public speaking or flying in airplanes; executives seek assertiveness training in order to become more effective with colleagues; lawyers go into psychoanalysis to control their "workaholism." There are long-term psychotherapy groups for people seeking to become more socially attractive or professionally desirable. Professional sports teams now have their own psychiatrists who regularly work with the players to improve their concentration, motivation, and communication.

To what degree are people who are simply unhappy turning themselves into patients, relabeling sorrow as "depression," anxiety as "post-traumatic stress disorder," trepidation as "adjustment disorder"? At what point along the spectrum are we medicalizing the human condition rather than treating psychopathology? The problem of grief and depression illustrates the dilemma, for it is difficult to know when a sorrowful and *sad person* should be declared a *depressed patient*. For some, grief becomes so intense and so prolonged that the bereaved person is diagnosed as having a psychiatric disorder, called a major depression. As many as 10 or even

20 percent of bereaved people (approximately 160,000 Americans) experience clinical depression such as this and are in need of professional treatment to help them through mourning. But how do we determine the point at which a parent's grief over the loss of a child goes beyond the expected sadness and despair and becomes pathological? Is it a disease when a widower of seventy-nine remains preoccupied with his wife for months following her death, after half a century of marriage? He finds that the little routines of daily life, such as the morning walk they used to take to the newsstand together, are no longer worth doing. He bursts into tears when he realizes that there is no one to tell about the latest episode of his favorite TV show. He is isolated, despondent, despairing, and wishing he were dead. But how are we to decide whether such a response is so extreme that it is abnormal, a pathological depression?

This dilemma arises because we now possess effective psychiatric techniques, new psychoactive drugs, new forms of family and behavioral therapy that enable us to help people with psychological problems we were never able to treat before. In dealing with painful emotional states, we encounter the same phenomenon we saw in dealing with maladaptive behavior and undesirable bodily characteristics: medical advances, combined with the universal wish to relieve our discomfort, have fueled a medicalization of affliction and suffering.

The Medical-Industrial Complex

Now let us look at several forces that have contributed to the medicalization of life and the expansion of patienthood. One of these is the commercialization of health. A giant "medical-industrial complex,"[35] which promotes a medical ideology and then translates it into consumer demand, has arisen. An alliance of advertisers, manufacturers, entrepreneurs, and advocacy groups have discovered that medicalization is lucrative. They promote the fantasy that good health can be purchased, and then they market products and services that are supposed to deliver us into the promised land of wellness.

Consumers are constantly reminded of the myriad threats to health, often by exaggeration of the risks involved, and then convinced of the necessity for products and services to protect them. Deeply submerged anxieties about disease and nutrition and physical appearance are first mobilized, and then channeled into consumer demand. Proprietary health-care corporations, advocacy groups, even hospitals seek to generate an appetite for health-related goods and services with hoopla, promotional buildup, and publicity. In order to stimulate demand and expand market share, people must be convinced of what they need and want. But in so doing, the medical-industrial complex creates a climate of alarm and a sense of omnipresent danger about health.

Once insecurity has been aroused, the way is clear for the peddling of panaceas to assuage it. Our anxieties can be harnessed to fuel burgeoning markets for exercise machines and fat farms, face-lifts and eyedrops, deodorants and vitamins. Chewing gum is sold as tooth polish, cereals are promoted as tonics. We are made to feel that our survival depends upon how wisely we choose from an array of products available to us. One trip down the drugstore aisle discloses remedies for every conceivable bodily state and sensation, for every vexation to which man is heir: stomach gas, stomach acidity, tired blood, tired eyes, yellow teeth, smoker's teeth, dandruff, athlete's foot, constipation, hemorrhoids, halitosis, and the rest. In pronouncements by "experts," and through advertisements and press conferences, the medical-industrial complex promotes the fantasy that anything disappointing about our bodies can be corrected, that every discomfort can be eliminated. A radio commercial for a group of plastic surgeons asks soothingly: "Is there anything about your face or body you are dissatisfied with? . . . Is your nose too long, your bust too large or too small?" This attitude appears in the popular press as well: "Women . . . want not only longer lives, but health and beauty too. With science as our handmaiden, we may yet achieve that Eden," says an article in the *Ladies Home Journal*.[36]

The result has been the transformation of health care from a necessity into a luxury, something we want and to which we feel entitled.[37] Medical care used to be sought only when necessary, when we were sick; now it is something for the healthy to avail themselves of as well, as part of a more general desire to feel good, to satisfy an appetite, to fulfill a wish.

The medical-industrial complex's motive is not obscure: it is financial, since unhealthy concerns can generate healthy profits. We thus find a wide array of organizations with vested interests in medicalizing society, including manufacturers and merchandisers, insurance companies, doctors and public-health departments, public-interest groups, and voluntary health associations. Prominent among them are the investor-owned medical-care corporations: for-profit hospitals and diagnostic laboratories, ambulatory surgery centers and "health stops," and home health-care services. It is estimated that they garner one-quarter of the total amount of money spent on personal health care, so the profits to be made here are enormous.[38]

Hospitals have been among the quickest to commercialize. Many have undertaken aggressive public-relations campaigns, and advertising by hospitals was estimated to be $1 billion in 1986.[39] They boast elective surgery at convenient hours and entice customers with gourmet food and free transportation. They have opened retail shops and catering services, and they offer frequent-user bonuses patterned after the airlines' frequent-flyer programs.[40] Saint Joseph Medical Center in Burbank, California, advertises a new device for treating kidney stones with the line "Kidney stones? Who Ya Gotta Call . . . Stonebusters!"[41] One advertisement, proposed but never run, read "Mikhail Gorbachev knows how lasers can be used to zap enemy missiles. But he might be surprised to learn how they can also be used to zap away problem birthmarks, like the reddish-purple one on his forehead."[42]

Industries outside of the medical-industrial complex have also found medicalization profitable. The food industry, increasingly concentrating upon "health" foods, is a good example. Though this category is difficult to define, ranging from whole-wheat pizza to low-salt tonic water, it has been estimated that health- and fitness-conscious food consumers spent almost $26 billion in 1983, mostly for reduced-calorie, reduced-fat, and high-fiber foods. Sales of these "healthy" products are climbing at the rate of 6 percent a year; major corporate executives call this the biggest trend in the food industry in half a century.[43]

Advertising campaigns emphasize the health implications of products only remotely related to health, linking every imaginable item to illness or wellness. Swimming-pool companies, for example, court buyers by noting that they make pools for the handicapped and for those "allergic" to chlorine. Real-estate developers promote their condominiums' location as being "within minutes of a major medical center." Cellular telephones are advertised as healthful because they reduce the stress of being stuck in traffic and unable to conduct business.

Even the nonprofit, voluntary health associations and charities, such as the American Cancer Society, the American Heart Association, and the Easter Seals Society, have a stake in calling our attention to health and disease. They raise funds for research and treatment of particular diseases, and at the same time mount educational campaigns to alert the public to their dangers. In the race for funding, each organization must compete with the others to sustain public concern about "their" disease. Each thus tends to amplify its message about research and treatment needs.[44] While their public-service announcements fill the airwaves, they meet the public clamor for assistance with telephone hotlines, some with catchy toll-free numbers, for problems from acne (the "Acne Help Line" at 800-235-ACNE) to digestive disorders (the "Gutline") to hearing problems (800-222-EARS).

The Health Fair is a commercial event that epitomizes the medicalized 1980s. Health fairs are staged almost weekly somewhere in the nation by private companies, promoters, and entrepreneurs. While such fairs might have attracted 500 people a decade ago, they now rival car and boat shows, drawing as many as 17,000.[45] Things that we considered flaky only recently, such as inversion tables, ion showers, and foot-massage techniques, now find a wide audience. Electric hospital beds are sold for use at home by people who are well, because their "orthopedic design" promises "healthier sleep." The replacement of bedroom furniture with hospital furniture graphically depicts the seepage of medical products and medical images into daily life.

Support for the Sick

An important social trend going hand-in-hand with medicalization is the decline in traditional sources of support for the sick. As the expression and management of distress have increasingly been channeled into the medical arena, religious buttresses have crumbled, and family care of the sick has been eroded by the decline of the extended family. And where are we to find consolation for suffering and affliction if not in church or at home?

Secularizing Sickness

Religious belief helps people bear suffering, and religious rituals support patients and families as they cope with sickness and death. Traditional religion buffers illness by counseling fatalism and resignation to the will of God. Sickness and pain are interpreted as necessary. Thus Buddha's First Noble Truth is "Life is suffering." (Interestingly, the necessity of suffering is also a central feature of mystical religions and of many atheist philosophies such as Stoicism as well.)

The belief in a hereafter provides solace and helps us to minimize the cruelties of this earthly life. As difficult and painful as life seems, it is comforting to know that what happens here on this earth is unimportant in the larger scheme of things. The best is yet to come; death holds out the promise of another world, a world in which suffering ends.

In addition, when illness is perceived as a part of God's plan for humankind—as His will—then there is a context in which to endure, dignify, and even to value suffering.[46] The most tormenting illness is not totally meaningless, capricious, and unjust: it is God working his way in the world. Suffering acquires a certain value because it is an offering to God, a redemptive test of our faith, a sacrifice we make for Him. Thus religious belief comforts the sick by providing a rationale for suffering.

Beyond the solace of belief, religious institutions and religious rituals in and of themselves provide comfort and mitigate suffering. Churches and other religious institutions, prayer and healing rites, hearten us and help us to cope. Religious settings and functions allow us to commiserate with and console the sick. They inculcate forbearance, patience, resignation, and self-control. And they also help us tolerate pain and disability by marshaling support for the sick person and his family.[47]

In sixteenth- and seventeenth-century Protestant England, the appropriate response to an accident or illness was to search one's soul for moral error. Although disease obeyed natural laws, it was believed to be sent by God to punish sin.[48] Thus, the ultimate power to regain one's health resided not in the individual, but in God and in the relationship the sick person had with God. Man could influence his health only indirectly, by performing righteous and devout acts.

But since the eighteenth century in America, illness has increasingly been viewed as a secular event. Rationalist and then scientific ideas about disease have gradually gained ascendency over the theological view of illness.[49] We now regard sickness as a natural phenomenon whose occurrence has nothing to do with religious, magical, or moral forces. The *Physicians' Desk Reference* has supplanted the Holy Bible in the bedside table drawer.

As religious medicine has declined, the healing and coping functions of religion are assumed more and more by medical personnel and medical institutions. Today, healthcare professionals increasingly offer pastoral services. Social workers, visiting nurses, therapists, and other paramedical personnel assist families in mourning, arrange for the daily needs of the disabled, and provide home care. The strength that people used to find in church may now be sought in a therapeutic support-group meeting at a hospital.

As sickness has become a more secular experience, the redemptive aspects of suffering and the rationale for bearing it are lost, and it is harder to find solace and support when disease strikes.* Sickness becomes more dreadful and more terrifying, and we face it more alone and more naked. Without religious meaning, it is devoid of consolation, for it is not going to bring the sufferer a sense of virtue or salvation, or even necessarily bring him closer to his fellow parishioners.

In sum, we've come to worry more about our health as we worry less about our souls; we focus upon spiritual pain less as we focus upon bodily pain more; as we lose the comforting notion of immortality, the tension about our mortality rises.

---

* It is interesting to note, in this regard, that community surveys of symptom reporting show that the less active a person's religion, the more bodily symptoms he reports being troubled by.[50]

The Decline in Domestic Care

There has been another, complementary, social movement. It is the decline in domestic medicine and in the family as a source of care. The breakup of the extended family has depleted our most critical resource for coping with sickness and suffering. More and more often, there is no one to care for us when we get sick, to help us to function with chronic disability, to support us and comfort us when we are in pain.

In earlier times, most of the care of the sick took place within the family. But with urbanization, industrialization, and increasing geographic mobility, the extended family broke up, leaving fewer relatives close by in case of illness. The large, extended family has been replaced by a smaller, nuclear family, and the number of unattached individuals living alone has risen, particularly in cities. Simultaneously, the number of flexible, expandable households that take in nonfamily members as boarders and lodgers has declined.[51] In addition, in the last decade or two, the size of the nuclear family itself has shrunk as couples have fewer children. The proportion of households composed of six or more people has therefore been cut in half between 1970 and 1983, and more than one-fifth of American households now consist of one person living alone, a shift particularly evident in the rising numbers of elderly widows.

Domestic care has also been undermined by greater instability of the family unit. Divorce rates have risen: for people marrying in the 1980s, the risk of divorce exceeds 50 percent. Along with this, the proportion of single-parent families continues to increase. Our view of marriage has shifted to stress the intensity of sexual ties, seeing it more as a "relationship" and less as an "institution."[52] Thus, even the small family units that do exist are often fragile and impermanent.

These changes in family structure and in residential patterns have been accompanied by a shift in the locus of medical care from the family to professional practitioners, hospitals, and clinics.[53] This shift is particularly obvious in the chronic care of the elderly, who increasingly are looked after in the medical-care system or in community institutions with medical supervision, such as nursing homes and "life care" communities. With the dissolution of the system of family support, isolated people increasingly seek out physicians for support, advice, and the opportunity to express their feelings. They turn to medical institutions in lieu of family for simple interpersonal contact, a sense of belonging, and assistance in coping with a variety of life's stresses and tribulations.

Medicalization Can Amplify Distress

Situation and circumstance affect the way we each think about our health and how healthy we feel. We have seen several aspects of contemporary American culture that cause us to assess our health more negatively by providing a disturbing context for that assessment. First, in medicalizing more and more of life, we have come to think of many distressing, and even some normal, characteristics as disorders which might be treatable. Second, powerful commercial forces heighten our health fears while simultaneously suggesting that medical care should not be a matter only of need but also of desire. And finally, the decline of religious and family resources for coping with illness makes it more fearsome.

The growth of medicine's diagnostic and therapeutic power is one of our greatest triumphs. Preventive medicine and diagnostic screening save lives and obviate untold suffering. The discovery that alcoholic liver disease, poor school performance, or interpersonal aggression can each be a symptom of a treatable disorder is a profound advance. The disfigured accident victim, the infertile couple, and the woman disabled before each menstrual period may now be helped in ways that were not possible even a few years ago. Likewise, modern psychiatric treatment is effective for many who are deeply troubled by psychiatric disorders.

But medicalization is a two-edged sword. Along with its benefits, medicalization produces a sort of loss of innocence, heightening our concern about our health even while we remain well: we now know about future illnesses we are at risk for, and we are acutely aware of the possibility of having an occult disease that has not yet announced its presence with symptoms. While going to the doctor more frequently can mean better medical care, it can also mean amplifying minor disorders and the wear and tear of life, states that would be better regarded with forbearance as nuisances to be minimized rather than as serious diseases to be worried about and attended to. Closer medical scrutiny leads to closer self-scrutiny and a heightened sensitivity to bodily dysfunction and discomfort, as we saw in chapter 2. Medical advances call our attention to all of our uncomfortable physical and mental experiences, since it is possible that they represent some new disorder we have just learned to detect and treat. Medicalization can make undesirable physical characteristics feel like deformities and lead us to imagine that every vexation has a diagnosis and every affliction a treatment.

The very act of being diagnosed, of learning that you have a disorder you didn't know about, can have a negative impact on physical and psychological well-being. Simply being told that you have a disease, even when it causes no symptoms and no treatment is undertaken, itself produces disability and psychological distress. Studies of asymptomatic people with high blood pressure have shown that merely learning of their disorder results in more absenteeism from work, increased psychological symptoms, and greater dissatisfaction with marriage and home life.[54]

Another danger of medicalization is that it stimulates unrealistic fantasies that whatever ails us is curable. Thinking of maladaptive behavior as a disease seduces us into hoping that we might one day be able to treat human foibles such as stupidity or cruelty. But incompetence and criminal behavior can never be treated out of existence, no matter how much we learn about the subtle brain diseases that make people prone to violence or addictions or slow to learn. Not all deviant or maladaptive behavior is pathological. Similarly, there is much physical discomfort, like fatigue and indigestion and headaches, that is not caused by disease. The fact of the matter is that these are inherent features of life, and they cannot be "treated" or "cured." Medicalization, however, makes us *imagine* that all discomfort is remediable, rather than something that must be coped with and endured. This attitude appears to be at the heart of the current epidemic of illicit drug use. Believing that we don't really have to put up with life's limitations and discomfort, believing that a remedy must exist, we treat ourselves with a pill, a snort, a toke, or even a shot.

Our stunning medical successes should not blind us to the ultimate limitations of biomedical progress. This may seem like a bit of a straw man, but recent history reveals highly exaggerated fantasies of what science and technology can accomplish, and there is a prevalent cultural myth that sickness and suffering, as broad categories of human experience, will one day surrender to medical advance. As we shall see later, when such fantasies are not borne out, there can be an unintended deleterious impact upon our subjective feelings of health.

CHAPTER 7

Beliefs: As You Sow, So Shall You Reap

WE NOW TURN to some prevalent beliefs that are important in understanding our contemporary preoccupation with health and disease. In discussing the psychology of health in chapter 2, we discovered that the thoughts a person has about his health—his information, ideas, and opinions—shape his sense of physical well-being. It is in this context that we look at some of our society's most salient beliefs about health. These are not facts but widespread, albeit subliminal, ideas that may not be expressed in so many words, but that nevertheless influence how we live, what we say, and how we behave.

Health Through Self-Control and Willpower

Many of us believe that we have acquired the power to control our health. With the proper exercise of our mental faculties, prudent behavior, and the miracles of modern biomedicine, we think we can ensure our survival. It's the quintessential American ideal: you can achieve almost anything if you put your mind to it and work hard enough for it. While we used to express this ideal in terms of social aspiration (anyone can grow up to be a millionaire or to be President), we now express it in terms of corporeal aspiration as well, believing that we can determine our own medical destiny.

Our advertisements, the health themes in magazines and books, the concept of wellness, the cult of the healthy lifestyle reveal this ideology of control, this sense of personal efficacy about health. More than a third of the respondents to a *Psychology Today* national survey are firmly convinced that what they do to stay healthy really counts. The ideology is revealed, for instance, in the testimonials of those who believe that a strong will to live has saved them from a fatal disease, and in the doctrine of holistic health. "Health and happiness *can* be ours if we desire; we can create our personal reality, down to the finest detail," says a holistic-medicine practitioner in his introduction to *The Holistic Health Handbook.*[1]

A positive mental outlook, good nutrition and physical conditioning, self-care, abstinence from alcohol and cigarettes are not only supposed to keep us from getting sick, but even to retard aging and delay death. A television commercial touting a high-fiber cereal for its value in preventing colon cancer concludes with the satisfied cereal-lover cooing reassuringly, "It's nice to know there are things I can do." If we do the rights things, like avoiding stress, buckling our seat belts, and obtaining regular checkups, then we will stay healthy. We must examine ourselves conscientiously: breasts, testicles, stool testing for occult blood, and, of course, skin, to check for skin cancer. *Prevention* magazine advises: "Examine your birthday suit on your birthday . . . Don't ignore your moles . . . keep tabs on them. . . . All you need is a full-length mirror, a good light, and the cooperation of a family member or friend."[2] In order for us to detect the early transformation of a benign mole into a malignant melanoma, the magazine suggests that once a year we measure every mole with a ruler and record it on a drawing of our body. A spouse or friend helps by cataloging "the moles in the hard-to-see areas." And the lucky recipient is coached to "return the favor on the other's birthday."

Good health is not a gift, not mere good luck, not the

product of heredity or of regular everyday activities. Rather, it is the result of conscious, goal-directed behavior. Will-power, resolve, and unwavering dedication to the goal are necessary. Research interviews have revealed that when people talk of threats to their health, their understanding of health, and prescriptions for maintaining health, they speak of self-discipline, self-control, and willpower.[3] Beyond intention, good health requires sustained hard work. Health maintenance is thought to be a matter of abstaining from things we enjoy and denying our natural proclivities toward dangerous habits. Put down those cigarettes, pass up the whipped cream, shut off the television and do some sit-ups. With perseverence and a strict regimen of restraint and denial, health can be achieved and preserved indefinitely.[4]

The themes of self-discipline and self-control, of abstention and renunciation as health imperatives, are apparent in our attitudes toward body weight.[5] Obesity is seen as evidence of poor self-control and weakness and letting yourself go. It suggests you are self-indulgent, impulsive, and lazy. Thinness, on the other hand, is an unmistakable sign that you have discipline, willpower, and self-control.[6] Dieting is seen as a form of self-discipline, a healthy assertion of self-mastery. Losing weight is admired because it means having renounced powerful appetites and urges.[7] Historically, fasting has been a way to demonstrate control over the demands of the flesh, and people who fasted, like religious ascetics, often described experiencing a powerful sense of virtue. Nowadays, many patients with anorexia nervosa likewise report that ascetic gratification comes from starving themselves.[8]

"Healthy habits" and the "healthy lifestyle" have come to be seen as moral and virtuous, as standards for judging character and personal worth. And if health-promoting behavior is moral, then illness may be the result of moral failure or lapse. Failing to live a healthy lifestyle connotes neglect, sloth, and lack of self-respect. If we fail to revere our bodies, then we deserve censure.[9] Being ill means being guilty. For example, a perfectly healthy medical outpatient noted, "I'm really kind of angry at myself for not getting more exercise—it's almost like a weakness that I can't make myself do it. And I know it's good for you. Maybe I'm just somebody without willpower."

In a similar case, a nun undergoing treatment for a degenerative neurological disease found the weakness in her leg progressing much more rapidly. At her regular appointment with her neurologist, she could not bring herself to tell him of her worsening symptoms because she suspected they resulted from her failure to adhere to the exercise regimen he had prescribed, and she didn't want him to think she was lazy. Soon after, when she became feverish, she went to the emergency room at a different hospital so that her physician would not know she had sought medical attention. There she was actually relieved to learn that her symptoms were caused by a urinary-tract infection and not by her failure to take good care of her body.

This ideology of control over health has another important consequence. Our subjective feeling of healthiness is adversely affected if we are not doing all the things we are supposed to do to stay healthy. The failure to carry out these normative health practices itself can make us feel unhealthy, even though we may be entirely well.[10] Thus a typical respondent in a research interview said: "Where I feel that I am not particularly healthy, perhaps, is maybe just in the consciousness that everyone seems to be going through now about health—jogging, not smoking, all of this. I am not really doing any of that and so I am concerned. . . ."[11]

Finally, if health is to be tied so closely to one's behavior, if you are responsible for your illness, then why shouldn't you be responsible for your medical bill as well? Insurers have already begun to question whether self-induced illnesses (such as lung cancer in a smoker, or the brain concussion of a motorcyclist without a crash helmet, or a recreational skier's broken leg) should be excluded from coverage, since, they argue, the patient has brought the illness upon himself.

The Increase in Behaviorally Caused Deaths

There are some good reasons for subscribing to the doctrine that we control our health by controlling our behavior, since in reality there *are* a number of ways in which we can influence health. There is a growing incidence of behavior-related causes of death. As a society we are doing unhealthy things, such as consuming harmful products, polluting the environment, pursuing high-risk activities, growing sedentary, and becoming addicted to harmful substances. Altering such behavior would indeed improve our health.

The illnesses most likely to kill us today differ in this way from those that killed our predecessors. In 1900 the three most frequent causes of death were all infections: pneumonia and influenza, tuberculosis, and gastrointestinal infections. And two of the next seven killers were infectious as well—kidney infections and diphtheria. There was little you could do at that time to protect yourself from these common killers.

Nowadays, however, we are not so often the passive victims of uncontrollable infectious agents. By 1980, heart disease was the most common cause of death, followed by cancer, strokes, accidents, and chronic lung disease, in that order. Cirrhosis of the liver was the eighth most frequent killer, and suicide was the tenth.* Behavior plays a role in each of these disorders. We can diminish the risk of heart disease by modifying diet and exercise; we can hope to escape lung cancer by not smoking; we can reduce the likelihood of suffering a stroke by adhering to a treatment regimen for hypertension; we can avoid cirrhosis of the liver by

---

* Influenza and pneumonia together constituted the sixth most common cause of death and were the only infectious diseases in the top ten. Diabetes was seventh, and atherosclerosis was ninth.

moderating our drinking. (AIDS is obviously another disease that can have a major behavioral component.)

Accidents and suicide, the fourth and tenth most common causes of death respectively, are of course the most behavior-related deaths of all. In 1983 there were 47,000 deaths in motor-vehicle accidents, 27,000 suicides, and more than 20,000 homicides. This self-destruction and violence is especially alarming among the young. It accounts for three-quarters of all deaths in the fifteen-to-twenty-four-year-old age group. The suicide rates for children and young adults tripled between 1950 and 1977, so that suicide has become the third leading cause of death in these groups. Homicide is now the most common cause of death for black males between fifteen and forty-four years of age. Almost one out of every 100 black youths who turned fifteen in 1983 will have been murdered by the age of twenty-four.[12]

Even when we examine infant and childhood death, we find that behavior is important. Deaths in the first year of life are most frequently attributable to congenital abnormalities, low birth weight, and prematurity. Though these are not the direct result of maternal behavior, a number of maternal behavioral risk factors predispose infants to these conditions. Maternal smoking and heavy alcohol use, for example, have each been associated with prematurity and lower infant birth weight. Poor maternal nutrition, drug abuse, and lack of regular prenatal care also predispose to them.

We have so far only considered the impact of behavior on mortality, but it also contributes mightily to morbidity. The bronchitis and chronic lung disease that result from smoking, veneral diseases, nonfatal automobile accidents and burns, the many medical consequences of drug and alcohol abuse merely hint at the role of unhealthy behavior in chronic illness and disability. Thus, the belief that we can control our health has a certain legitimacy: while we cannot determine the outcome of the game, or when it will end, we can to some degree stack the odds in our favor.

Self-Treatment:
The "Private Practice" of Medicine

Our belief in the personal control of health means an expansion of the duties and responsibilities we have as patients. When we are sick, there is more for us to do now than there used to be. When we leave the doctor's office, we can't forget about our illness until the next visit, because we are expected to assume the ongoing, day-to-day responsibility for our own medical management. The modern patient diagnoses and treats himself, a task requiring considerable knowledge and effort. In order to assume this supervisory and executive role, it is first necessary to do your homework, which entails reading about your condition in one of a number of new medical textbooks written for a lay audience, such as *The Columbia University College of Physicians and Surgeons Complete Home Medical Guide*. This new role for the patient leads to the not uncommon sight at our hospitals of patients in doctors' waiting rooms reading not *National Geographic,* but *The Annals of Internal Medicine* or *The New England Journal of Medicine.*

As modern patients, we are not passive recipients of the doctor's ministrations, vessels into which the doctor pours his elixirs. Rather, we are ancillary care-givers, a sort of apprentice physician, clinicians who monitor our own status and make treatment decisions. We therefore learn to regard our own bodies with clinical detachment, observing, testing, measuring, and examining them, just as a radiologist does when he scans an X ray or a surgeon does when he examines "an" abdomen. Thus there are moments when we think of ourselves as the doctor does, not just as a *person with* diabetes (to pick one example), but as a *case of* diabetes.

Two factors have fostered the development of this new executive role for patients: new technologies, and the self-help and self-care movements. People have always treated themselves extensively with traditional remedies, patent medicines, and folk nostrums. In the 1920s, for instance, 16 percent of the average family's medical expenditures were for patent medicines.[13] What is new to our era is the nature of the products that are available for self-treatment. For years, the thermometer was the only self-diagnostic device we had. If you had high blood pressure, it was checked by the doctor; if you suspected you were pregnant, a physician administered a pregnancy test. But now if you have hypertension you monitor your blood pressure, and if diabetic you determine your own blood-sugar level. There are kits for detecting pregnancy and diagnosing bowel cancer. If you have a urinary-tract infection you can test to see whether a course of antibiotics has cured you. Soon, home computers and interactive software will provide step-by-step guidance and supervision in these and other sorts of self-diagnosis and self-treatment. This variety of medical kits and tests available without a prescription, for use at home, make possible the "private practice" of medicine (as *Time* magazine calls it).

The sales of these products are booming. In 1984, revenues from home health-care kits totaled about $800 million,[14] and one manufacturer, Warner-Lambert, estimates that this market will grow 27 percent annually for the next five years.[15] An industry magazine has suggested that home medical-care devices will eventually be as common as wristwatches.[16] These new personal-health-care products turn each of us into a paramedic, acting out the doctrine of personal efficacy over health.

The self-care and self-help movements exemplify our increasing personal responsibility for medical treatment. Their fundamental aim is the acquisition of medical competence by the individual. Activities include disease prevention, coping with chronic disease, and acquiring diagnostic and treatment expertise, for example, learning to perform such techniques as breast self-examination and cardiopulmonary resuscitation. A cascade of national self-help associations has been generated, which now includes organizations for the sufferers of such rare diseases as Tay-Sachs disease and such common ones as psoriasis, as well as organizations for compulsive gamblers, midgets, and mothers of twins, to name but a few.

The self-care movement originally had political overtones of opposition to organized medicine and suspicion of medical professionals.[17] It began with the 1960s' counterculture attacks on psychiatry in books such as *The Myth of Mental Illness* and *One Flew Over the Cuckoo's Nest,* and on obstetrics and gynecology in *Our Bodies, Ourselves.* Feminists accused obstetricians and gynecologists of insensitivity to women's concerns and asserted that sexism and oppression were prominent in medical practice. They emphasized the woman's right to make decisions about her own body and the importance of learning to examine herself and provide gynecological self-care. We have seen this same fusion of heightened health consciousness, self-care, and feminism before, in a period that bore many similarities to our own.

In the first half of the nineteenth century, Jacksonian America entered a period of geographic mobility, rapid industrialization, and political upheaval. Beginning in the 1830s and 1840s, a popular health movement arose, partly in response to this social turmoil and rapid change. When it seemed that there was little the individual could do to control the massive social, political, and economic upheaval, people sought something that they could control. And many thought they found it in health.[18]

Then as now, the popular health movement had two prominent elements: feminism and self-care. Facing drastic changes in their role in the home and in the nature of the family, women seized upon health as an issue. They championed a movement that emphasized healthy personal habits and practices more than cure of disease by physicians. And as in the current era, they advocated self-care and the education of family members to recognize and take care of many illnesses in the home with the help of instructional courses and new manuals written for the purpose.[19]

The contemporary interest in alternative healing also reflects a waxing belief in personal efficacy over health. The holistic health movement emphasizes the emotional, mental, and spiritual aspects of health and illness, aspects over which the individual has control. Holism is oriented toward health promotion and disease prevention, maintaining that habits, attitudes, expectations, the way we work and live, and the ways we think and feel can make us sick or well. It encourages people to become active participants in the healing process and to take responsibility for their health.

Psychologizing Disease

Perhaps taking a cue from holistic healers, our society in general has come to believe in the healing power of the mind, in the control of health not just through behavior but through attitude, thought, and emotion. There is a deeply held societal conviction that mind and body are intimately linked in physical disease. We treat physical illness by doing something for the mind (for example, meditation, guided mental imagery, stress reduction, or relaxation training) and mental illness by doing something for the body (massage, exercising, nutritional therapies, or dance therapy). "Pain is the soul calling for help," says the owner of a stress-reduction center, expressing the view that physical distress ultimately has psychological roots.[20]

Attitude is thought to be especially important in coping successfully with many chronic disorders, enabling us to convert our illness into a positive "growth experience," or even to cure it. Norman Cousins, in his best-seller *Anatomy of an Illness,* reports curing himself of a severe disorder by adopting a healthy mental outlook, cultivating his sense of humor by watching comedy movies and reading humorous books, and taking vitamin C. Many people believe psychological treatments are an important adjunct to medical treatment. The search is on for more techniques like guided mental imagery, meditation, motivational exercises, and "mind development," all of which are intended to teach us how to "communicate" better with our bodies.

The yearning to find psychological explanations for physical diseases runs deep. Susan Sontag noted that a physical illness seems less real if it can be considered a "mental" event, because this suggests that we can *choose* not to be sick or to die. Psychologizing undermines the reality of the disease by providing an illusion of control over it. At its root, she feels this tendency to psychologize is a kind of spiritualism, an affirmation of the primacy of "spirit" over matter.[21]

In particular, a great deal of attention has been focused upon the role of the psyche in the long-term survival of cancer. It is believed that an upbeat attitude, a fighting spirit, and a strong will to live, especially when combined with the free and open expression of feelings of anger and distress, can help to cure cancer. In 1985, *The New England Journal of Medicine* published a study showing that psychological attitudes did *not* affect the progression of advanced cancers. More cheerful patients had no greater success than depressed ones in fighting their cancers, and pessimists were not more likely to die from recurrences than were optimists.[22] An editorial in the same issue raised broad questions about the effectiveness of positive thinking in fighting disease in general and was critical of psychological treatments for cancer. The editorial concluded, "It is time to acknowledge that our belief in disease as a direct reflection of mental state is largely folklore."[23] Most interesting from our viewpoint is not this conclusion itself, but the public outcry it generated. The editorial ignited a furor, eliciting as much mail as *The Journal* had ever received on any article it had published. The editor commented on this response: "I've been astonished by the intensity of the debate. It's as though I had attacked motherhood and happiness. People seem to want to believe that how we think matters for our health— that we have the power to control things that are powerful and frightening—but it's like doing a rain dance."[24]

If we credit courage and optimism for cure and survival, then we may also be implying fault when the outcome is less happy. If we can make ourselves healthy with positive thinking, then poor health must result from negative thoughts, or a failure to express repressed feelings or become more assertive. As a respondent in a survey put it, "You don't catch a cold, you succumb to it." If this is so, the patient whose disease progresses or spreads may feel guilty as well as ill. Just as we feel guilty for not pursuing a healthy lifestyle or following our treatment regimen, we can feel guilty for having the wrong attitude. The danger here is of heaping moral and personal condemnation on top of illness, of blaming the victim: "It's his own damn fault." Such an attitude is apparent in some of the holistic-health literature: "We choose our sickness when, through neglect or ignorance, we allow it to spread within us."[25] Falling ill is a failure, ascribed to an unwillingness to be well or an unconscious desire to be sick. As another writer states, "The only tyrant you face is your own inertia and absence of will—your belief that you are too busy to take your own well-being into your own hands and that the pursuit of self-health through a wellness-promotive lifestyle is too hard, complicated, or inconvenient.[26] Dr. Marcia Angell, an editor of *The New England Journal of Medicine,* pointed out what she considered an example of this sort of thinking in remarks made by the Humana Heart Institute's Dr. Allan Lansing. At a press conference Dr. Lansing expressed concern that artificial-heart recipient William Schroeder did not have the right attitude after his first stroke. Dr. Angell discerned the implication that Mr. Schroeder himself was responsible for the disappointing course of his treatment.[27]

Medical advances have nourished the psychologizing of disease just as they have nourished the other trends we've discussed. Biofeedback has opened up the possibility of attaining control over automatic bodily processes that we are not consciously aware of, such as the functioning of various organs. Physiological processes such as blood-vessel constriction, brain waves, and stomach contractions can be altered if people are provided with ongoing feedback about their moment-to-moment status. With such information, through trial and error we can learn to increase the flow of blood to a particular region of the body, lower blood pressure, or alter our brain waves. All of this fuels the fantasy that the control of the body can be reduced to mental terms and confers an expanded sense of personal efficacy.

The burgeoning field of psychoimmunology likewise stimulates the fantasy that we are on the threshold of controlling physical health with our mental faculties. Research has disclosed that the immune system is in fact influenced by life stresses (such as bereavement and unemployment) and emotional states (including helplessness and anxiety). Such research, which links psychological factors to the immune response, makes it seem as if disease resistance could ultimately be brought under conscious control. Because we want so fervently to believe this is true, we tend to exaggerate the strength of the link between the psyche and immune system and jump to the conclusion that we have the capability of controlling disease with thought, motivation, and attitude.

Stress

There is another way in which we believe we control our medical destiny. It is by regulating which life events we subject ourselves to and by curbing our reaction to them. "Stress" is public enemy number one. In nationwide polls, 89 percent of American adults report experiencing high levels of stress. Fully 59 percent say they feel great stress at least once a week.[28] Our patterns of medication consumption offer testimony to the fearsome power we endow it with: the three best-selling drugs in the United States are Tagamet for ulcers, Propranalol for high blood pressure, and valium for anxiety.

To many people, *stress* refers to the trivial hassles and pressures that we undergo every day. We know them by their symptoms: the sweating and the clenched jaw when someone zips into a parking space we were waiting for; the pounding heart while trying to make a tight plane connection. It's waiting in lines, filling out forms, having someone owe you money. As the poet Charles Bukowski wrote, "It's not the large things that send a man to the madhouse . . . no, it's the continuing series of small tragedies that send a man to the madhouse. . . . Not the death of his love but a shoelace that snaps with no time left."[29] To others, stress means major life events and crises that necessitate a change in our daily pattern: joblessness, problems with our children, divorce, legal troubles, financial difficulties.

Both types of stress have one thing in common, we believe; they make us sick by upsetting us emotionally. Stressful situations and events make us feel helpless, demoralized, or frustrated, and this frame of mind is unhealthy and pathogenic, the reasoning goes. So in the popularly held view, it is not just the stressful event that is significant, but our emotional response to it as well. Different people have very different emotional experiences of the same event. A snowstorm is stressful to the businessman late for an appointment across town, but not to the skier. One mother feels lonely and bereft when her daughter marries, while another is relieved and triumphant. As important as the nature of our trials and tribulations, it seems to us, is how we cope with them. People try to combat stress by preparing themselves mentally for it, by doing something physical to relieve it, or by altering their behavior so that they avoid stressful situations.[30] By coping better with stress, we believe we lessen our risk of physical illness.

Stressful life events do in fact have a deleterious impact upon general health. The relationship between unemployment, for example, and health status, is striking. For each 1 percent rise in unemployment, there are 1.9 percent more deaths from heart disease, 4.1 percent more suicides, and 3.3 percent more admissions to state mental hospitals.[31] Evidence suggests that stress is a significant factor in many psychosomatic diseases, including ulcers, high blood pressure, and asthma. More recently, we have begun to suspect that stress may affect one's vulnerability to infectious disease and even the progression of some chronic and degenerative diseases.

The point here is that the concept of stress meshes with the popular doctrine that we can control our health by taking charge of our lives. We believe we can choose to avoid stressful situations, and we can control our reactions to them when they do arise. In a survey of *Psychology Today* readers, over and again, respondents noted how crucial it is to "avoid stress—be calm and don't worry,"[32] and they reiterated the importance of shunning "those things in life that make you nervous, angry, or unhappy." Thus we must cultivate a positive and easy-going attitude toward life; we must "manage" stress, prevent it from getting to us; it is a question of mind over matter, and our health depends upon it.

Looking Good:
If You Don't Like Your Body, Change It

The doctrine of control extends beyond disease to include the body. We think it possible to remake the human body, to alter physical appearance, to conform to our ideal. Americans are preoccupied with improving and transforming and perfecting the body, pumping it up and slimming it down, trimming it off and shaping it up, preening it and caring for it. Thus we have a popular movie, *Perfect,* whose central character is a female ex–Olympic swimmer who dedicates herself to developing a perfect body as an aerobics instructor. In what other era could a forty-five-year-old man, Remar Sutton, leave everything and move to the Bahamas for one year, with the sole purpose of transforming his body from a flabby 200 pounds into that of a muscle-man?[33] His successful transformation through biking, jogging, and bodybuilding attracted a wide audience via newspaper columns and a book and culminated in the sale of movie rights and a planned lecture tour.[34]

Many people exercise and work out for reasons of health, as we discussed at length in chapter 5. But many others pursue strenuous physical conditioning in order to remake their bodies. Skinny, 135-pound weaklings really do walk into health clubs and tell fitness trainers, "I want to get big." The Nautilus machine is a tool for laboriously and lovingly sculpting muscles. The tanned, trim, taut, toned body is a precious object d'art, a masterpiece that we create ourselves. The body is then treasured, meticulously inspected, and painstakingly maintained in peak condition, like a teenager's motorcycle. And like the adolescent strutting around on his bike, we flaunt our bodies to show off what our hard work has created.

Our pursuit of a youthful, beautiful, and glamorous appearance fuels an enormous beauty industry, a stampede on plastic surgeons' offices, and a mass convergence on the weight rooms and whirlpool baths of vacation resorts and health clubs devoted entirely to the care of the body. "Looking good" is a contemporary byword. Said Perry Ellis, the designer, "People today think you can buy good looks. People are enslaved to the cosmetics counter, fad diets, designer clothes."[35]

Cosmetic surgery in particular is an invitation to design a new body, to "create a new you." A thirty-two-year-old psychologist told *Time* magazine how he regarded cosmetic surgery: "I see it as a little investment in health, like owning an electric toothbrush."[36] Surgery is portrayed by doctors and patients alike as an active and adaptive way of coping with the aging process and with life's problems—a way to get over a divorce or the death of someone important. Move an eyebrow up a bit, put a cleft in your chin, smooth away those crow's feet. Advertisements suggest a smidgen of "same-day surgery" to extinguish an offending blemish, as if it were as easy as erasing a mustache that had been penciled on a photograph of a beautiful model.

We also control appearance with cosmetics. Beginning early in the twentieth century, the pursuit of beauty began to be portrayed as a scientific undertaking. Scientific and medical advances were thought to prefigure the not too distant time when science would conquer aging and divulge the secret of beauty itself.[37] This marked the advent of the commercial beauty industry in the United States, and the epoch of the great cosmetic entrepreneurs, such as Elizabeth Arden and Helena Rubinstein.[38] By 1910, the use of makeup was widespread. Since then, to be considered beautiful has increasingly involved the use of artificial means: cosmetics, hair curling and coloring, and the rest. More recently, we have blurred the distinction between reality and appearance. Cosmetic advertisements and the remarks of cosmetic industry executives and cosmetic users reveal the underlying, though false, notion that cosmetics do not simply alter the user's appearance, but actually produce anatomic change and thus change one's physiognomy from the inside out.[39]

Skin care is currently the hottest sector of the beauty industry. In 1985, consumers spent $1.2 billion for cleansers, creams, gels, and foams to make their skin healthy and glowing. This resulted in a healthy and glowing industry, with projected sales increases in 1986 of as much as 13 percent.[40] When heart surgeon Dr. Christiaan Barnard endorsed a line of "rejuvenating" skin care products, sales exceeded $5 million in less than two months. Ignored by these consumers is the reality that trying to alter the skin itself with these products is, as a prominent dermatologist told *Time* magazine, about as effective as "giving someone a blood transfusion by rubbing blood into the skin."[41]

The point here is that our wishes for personal efficacy

extend beyond health and disease to the body itself, to the belief that we can actually alter our anatomy through diet, physical conditioning, and cosmetics.

The Apotheosis of Medical Care

We believe not only in the control of health and appearance through behavior, attitude, and stress reduction; we also believe fervently in the power of biomedicine to cure disease, reverse disability, and prolong life. Most people, in fact, believe that medical science will develop miracle cures for *all* of our most lethal diseases before they themselves are afflicted by them. Seventy percent of the American public is certain that cures for heart disease, strokes, cancer, lung disease, *and* diabetes will be found before they die.[42]

In World War II and the years just following, the power of scientific discovery and technological innovation became evident. A vast increase in government support for medical research began, and the National Institutes of Health were created. The infusion of money and manpower bore spectacular fruit in the mid-1950s with the production of a vaccine against poliomyelitis, that most feared crippling disease of children. This stunning triumph of biomedical research nourished the dream that we could ultimately conquer all the diseases to which man is heir. That dream flourishes today. Technological marvels such as pacemakers and laser therapy capture the imagination of people around the world and inspire awe. Now the promise of artificial hearts and kidneys, and transplanted lungs and livers, suggests there will be a time when we will replace diseased and worn-out body parts as methodically and as routinely as we repair automobiles. Disease seems to us a technical problem, like landing a man on the moon, that can be solved if we only bring enough resources and effort and skill to it.

We acknowledge few limitations on the benefits of medical intervention. No amount of medical care is too much, and every intervention is thought to have at least some potential benefit. If some medical care is good, then more must be better. When it comes to public policy and national priorities, most Americans still believe that we spend too little, not too much, on health care.[43] Though we acknowledge that rising costs are a societal problem, the polls also show that as individuals each of us is unwilling to accept any limit on the amount or type of medical care that we personally receive.[44] A majority of the respondents in a Harris poll opposed any reduction in federal health programs,[45] and two out of three Americans believe that federal spending for health care should be increased.[46] Ninety percent of Americans even favor the continued development of the most expensive programs, such as organ transplantation.[47]

When it comes to the treatment of the sick individual, our faith in medical efficacy is so strong that we are willing to go to any length, literally to pay any price. Rarely is a procedure spared, or a treatment forgone, if it offers even the remotest possibility of prolonging life. People should not die without our having done everything medically possible. There is an irresistible urge to do *something,* fostered by our belief in the omnipotence of medicine.

The problem, however, is that often we are merely forestalling death and prolonging what is nothing more than biological subsistence. We sometimes keep human bodies alive with life-support systems long after the possibility of meaningful life—of personhood—has been exhausted. We are so adamant about deflecting, if not controlling, the disease process, that we do so even when it brings only a Pyrrhic victory. Machines keep organ systems functioning while the physician stands by, unable to preserve the person. Our life-sustaining technology in these cases is really only death-delaying. And support for this "pull out all the stops," "no holds barred" strategy is widespread. Thus there have been more and more challenges to the authority of families and doctors to withhold or withdraw treatment from the moribund. The government and the courts have also sought to remove the discretionary power from parents and physicians to decide how to treat severely handicapped newborns, even when treatment only delays an inevitable death or perpetuates an existence consumed with pain and devoid of human contact.

The British, in contrast, acknowledge the limitations of personal medical care.[48] They spend one-third to one-half as much per capita on medical care as we do. Per capita, Britain has 67 percent fewer physicians and one-fifth to one-tenth as many intensive-care-unit beds, and they perform only one-tenth as much coronary-artery surgery as we do.[49] Interestingly, however, these differences are not associated with great differences in life expectancy, and in general the quality of British medicine is felt to be roughly equivalent to ours.

It is routine in Britain to deny some patients beneficial, even lifesaving, medical care. Patients and their families are aware of resource constraints and accept them.[50] Most respect the judgment of their physicians when informed that they are not suitable candidates for some type of care. Patients find solace in the knowledge that all care of substantive value has been provided and don't insist on treatment that is of marginal benefit. An English physician summed up their attitude: "I think you should prolong life, but you should not prolong dying."[51] British patients do not, as many Americans would, sue the physician for malpractice if some expensive, heroic, or experimental medical technique or procedure is withheld. Here, if an intervention exists, then it is likely to be tried. Anything less from our medical system is unacceptable.

Beliefs as Amplifiers

The doctrine of personal control over health has some basis in reality. Altering personal habits *can* reduce our chances of dying from some of the most common killers. Becoming a more active and informed partner in the medical care process makes that care better. Self-help organizations are beneficial to people coping with chronic illnesses and to those with behavioral problems such as obesity and alcoholism and smoking. Recognizing and managing the stresses of modern life can help both body and psyche. And competent, timely medical care is the most obvious way of influencing health.

All of these do provide us with some measure of control over health. And finding steps that we can take to control a situation is the best way of coping with it. But beyond a point, we amplify the illness experience by expanding the sphere of personal responsibility so much. The mandate for self-discipline and self-control becomes so burdensome and so arduous that it begins to erode our sense of physical well-being and makes us feel increasingly insecure about health. Because in this new world of enhanced personal efficacy we know more about what we can do for our health, common and innocuous situations, emotions, and personal habits take on serious health implications and consequences, even if we are perfectly healthy at the time. And once we become sick, patienthood becomes more taxing and complicated because we are now deeply immersed in the treatment process. By becoming our own physicians, we have heaped all the physician's cares on top of all the cares of being ill and being a patient. Sickness becomes a testing ground for our character, our commitment to recovery, our ability to impose mind over matter. All of this amplifies the experience of illness by making it a more significant event, something to which we should devote more time and effort and attention. Thus while greater personal responsibility for, and control over, health leads to some objective benefits, it also makes the subjective illness experience more pervasive, arduous, and demanding.

The doctrine that we control our health can also amplify our infirmities and ailments in that in addition to getting old, getting sick, or succumbing to the ravages of a severe disease, the victim now has the added burden of suspecting that it happened because he was unmotivated, undisciplined, or neglectful. The belief in personal efficacy opens the door for disillusionment, blame, and self-reproach. The expectation that you can remake your body and your face, that the early discovery of cancer means you won't die of it, that biofeedback will eliminate chronic pain makes things worse when it turns out not to be true.

There is also another problem with the ideology of control over health. Believing that you can control something when you really can't makes it seem worse. And our sense of efficacy is excessive, because in large measure our biological fate does not lie in our hands. We cannot simply choose not to be ill. While we use the terms *health* and *medicine* interchangeably, as in "health-care providers," "health consumers," "health insurance," and "health-maintenance organization," the reality is that we cannot deliver health, or insure health, or provide or purchase health as if it were a commodity. The awful fact is that we cannot avoid getting gallstones or arthritis or glaucoma or a thousand other ailments, some trivial, some horrible. We cannot will ourselves into surviving cancer. Concealing the signs of aging with surgery and weight training is not the same as slowing the aging process, and cosmetics alter appearances, not reality. The fat person is not fat because he is lazy, and the person who suffers a second heart attack was not simply inadequately motivated after his first. There are limits to what medical care can accomplish. Our sphere of influence is actually rather limited when compared to the effects of heredity, environment, culture, and chance. Though we can transplant the human heart and restore vision painlessly with lasers, we cannot loosen arthritic fingers, make a palsied limb work again, or restore consciousness to a comatose brain, much less prevent athlete's foot or cure the common cold. In short, and as we've said before, though we may sometimes be able to stack the odds in our favor, we generally do not determine the outcome. It is still worth keeping your fingers crossed.

CHAPTER 8

Start Storing Your Own Blood: Our Mood of Dis-ease

THE HOLIDAY SEASON is approaching. On the wall of an elevator in a New Orleans hospital is a poster in serene shades of gray. It shows a delicate line drawing of a pastoral scene, a tranquil woman resting in a field of wildflowers. Beneath her is the soothing invitation, "Give her peace of mind for Christmas." The poster suggests a Christmas gift package consisting of a mammogram to detect breast cancer and a screening test for endometriosis. Has illness really become such a major source of unease? Like Frank Carson, with whom we opened the book, many of us worry about our health and find that the possibility of sickness is on our minds a lot. Good health seems a precarious and fragile state that can be maintained only with heroic effort, spartan discipline, and constant vigilance. We don't feel robust or hardy or vigorous, and we lack a feeling of physical well-being, a sense of security about our health and confidence about our bodies. Every bodily sensation is a source of concern, since we are told to monitor every heartbeat and every bowel movement and to seek a medical opinion for every ache. And even if we do happen to feel fine today, that is no guarantee that tomorrow will not bring the first sign of some dreaded disease. Rather than living exuberantly, we are timid and apprehensive, afraid of getting sick, easily thrown off track by minor infirmities, dismayed by the specter of advancing age.

Our Dis-ease About Disease

Our society acts as if it were perched on the brink of a medical catastrophe, while simultaneously denying that there is anything to be concerned about. Many of us regard health the way a self-made millionaire might regard his bounty: having vowed when he was poor to acquire great riches, he now finds himself unable to enjoy them for fear they will be stolen away. Eternally vigilant, afraid of losing what he has, he barricades himself in his house and stays awake through the night, watching out for burglars, guarding rather than enjoying his hard-earned treasures. As a society, rather than relishing our collective good health, we spend our time subduing the real and imaginary threats to it. And the more assiduously we try to guard our good health, the less confident and assured we become, and the less we are able to enjoy it.

This cultural climate of apprehension and anxiety nourishes the incipient hypochondriacal concerns that we all harbor to some degree; it leads us to amplify trivial symptoms and fosters a mood of exacting watchfulness when it comes to health. We must be careful lest life be reduced to a continuous vigil of diet, digestion, and excretion. We could become a nation of healthy invalids, crippled not by disease but by the idea of disease. As Lewis Thomas has written in *The Medusa and the Snail,* "The new danger to our well-being . . . is in becoming a nation of healthy hypochondriacs, living gingerly, worrying ourselves half to death. . . . We keep telling each other this sort of thing, and back it comes on television or in the weekly newsmagazines, confirming all the fears, instructing us, as in the usual final paragraph of the personal-advice columns in the daily paper, to 'seek professional help.' Get a checkup. Go on a diet. Meditate. Jog. Have some surgery. Take two tablets, with water. *Spring* water. If pain persists, if anomie persists, if boredom persists, see your doctor."[1]

Since we are constantly admonished that almost everything we consume, do, or interact with has health consequences, daily life provides fertile soil in which the obsession with health can take root. There is a sense that our health is in constant jeopardy, so that almost every decision we make becomes critical—buying shoes, for example. You must select shoes that are orthopedically correct, "engineered for the biomechanics of walking," in order to improve circulation, relieve stress, reduce body fat, and assure yourself of remaining "injury free."[2] Even more grave is the selection of our children's shoes: an advertisement for Stride Rite children's shoes discourages buying sneakers for children because, an orthopedist assures us, "on rugs, babies trip five times more often in sneakers than in shoes. Three times more often on tiles." How many cups of coffee have you had so far today? Did you floss your teeth last night? Is your weight creeping up this week? When was the last time your eyes were examined for glaucoma? If you keep very still while you check your resting pulse, you might just be able to hear your arteries hardening or your mitral valve clicking.

There is an endless cascade of new diseases to worry about. Endometriosis, for example: "Severe menstrual pain. It could be warning you of more pain ahead. . . . It may be a symptom of endometriosis—a condition that may affect up to 10 million women. Untreated, endometriosis can grow increasingly worse. . . ."[3] Or chlamydia: "Chlamydia: Silently devastating . . . the most common sexually transmitted disease . . . is nine times more widespread than herpes and more than twice as common as gonorrhea. . . . A leading cause of infertility . . . poses a greater health threat than physicians once believed."[4] And the old dangers are still around—scoliosis, for example: "Help screen your child for scoliosis: it's 30 seconds that could change your child's life"; and ileitis and colitis, which "can strike any one, any time"; and an enlarged prostate: "The prostate—ignore it at your peril."[5]

It is hard to keep up with the torrent of medical warnings,

an ever-lengthening list of do's and don'ts. Too little breakfast threatens longevity, while too much breakfast causes obesity. Too little calcium causes osteoporosis, but too much calcium causes kidney stones. Sedentary and inactive jobs cause heart attacks, while tense and competitive jobs cause high blood pressure. But don't quit work, because retirement is just as bad: feeling useless and undervalued can be fatal too. What could be safer than watching television at home? "Too much TV linked to obese youngsters," the Associated Press warns,[6] since it turns out that the more television a child watched, the more obese he is as a teenager.[7] What could be safer than sitting still? Yet *Prevention* magazine warns: "Caution: prolonged sitting may be hazardous to your health." "You can overdose on sitting," they inform us, recounting the dangers of back disease, varicose veins, and thrombophlebitis that result from sitting.[8]

Our dis-ease about disease is self-perpetuating. It fuels itself, each worry engendering two more, alarm leading to greater alarm. Like a ghastly rumor, our apprehension mushrooms to include more and more under its shadow. First our fears about our own health grew to encompass that of our children. When some researchers found evidence of atherosclerosis beginning in childhood, a series of articles in the popular press warned about seven-year-olds already marked with the risk factors for heart disease. Headlines advised screening young schoolchildren for elevated blood-cholesterol levels. Given this alarming picture, formal physical education classes at "junior gyms," beginning when the child was three months old, were advocated.[9]

The next alarm was sounded when we learned that our unhealthy habits jeopardized not only ourselves, but others around us as well. We'd known how unhealthy cigarette smoking is for the smoker himself, but now concern arose about the dangers of "passive" or "involuntary" smoking— the dangers of inhaling other people's cigarette smoke. Then we became concerned about the health of the unborn fetus as we realized the dangers of maternal behavior such as drinking and drug use. Now our concern for the unborn child has extended back to include maternal health practices *before* conception (so-called prepregnancy care), and we are told that the prospective mother must alter her health habits at least twenty-eight days *before* attempting to get pregnant. Even the prospective father should take special precautions before trying to have a baby: don't forget, *American Health* magazine warns, that "smoke gets in your sperm," and watch out for "steamed semen."[10]

Most recently, the health of our pets has fallen under our anxious scrutiny. In magazines and newspapers and on the radio, we are taught about pet diseases, the proper use of the veterinarian, how to practice preventive medicine on dogs and cats and even birds. There seems to be no end to the putative threats posed by disease. Our feeling of dis-ease is growing, there doesn't seem to be any sanctuary, and no one is safe—not our family, not innocent bystanders, not future generations, not even our pets.

Anxiety Fuels Our Symptoms

Our pervasive mood of apprehension and alarm about health is significant because, as we saw in chapter 2, anxiety is a potent amplifier of normal sensations and trivial dysfunctions, making them more intense and more disturbing until they seem to be the malignant symptoms of some dreaded disease. Night sweats, for example, have become a fearsome symptom in the public mind, since they can be associated with tuberculosis, lymphoma, and other cancers. Yet night sweats are common among healthy people and, as long as they are not accompanied by a fever, are rarely a sign of illness.[11] Most of us have always considered snoring to be benign, but now medical commentators recommend professional attention for snorers, warning that it erodes the quality of sleep and can be associated with angina and high blood pressure. "Desk jobs and colon cancer," "Diabetes strikes one out of every 20 Americans. No family is immune," "Are you getting too much radiation?" are typical of the alarms constantly being sounded in articles on health. Can you read through a magazine without wondering about your own symptoms and whether they might not be more ominous than you'd thought?

It is no surprise that practicing internists see increasing numbers of "worried well" patients. Some of them fear a specific disease, while others have vaguer concerns and seek, quite literally, "a clean bill of health." And when the physician's search discloses nothing wrong, many then worry that their diagnostic workup was not thorough enough. Asymptomatic men in their twenties request electrocardiograms, and patients with headaches obviously caused by tension are not satisfied until a CAT scan has been performed. "People almost seem to be primed to fear the worst, meaning cancer or AIDS, and it doesn't take much—maybe somebody famous dying, or an acquaintance getting ill—to set them into a panic that they too have a silent and undiscovered but life-threatening illness," observes a busy internist at an academic medical center.

As one observer said, "There must be something the matter with someone who goes to see a doctor when there is nothing the matter with him." Why do people spend money and take time to go to the doctor when they are well? A healthy twenty-two-year-old registered nurse visited her internist saying she had just discovered a lump in her breast. She had been working on a cancer floor at a large hospital, and the work was hard for her. This was partly because many of the patients referred to her hospital were especially difficult cases, "the worst horror stories," as she put it. She got to know her patients and took it hard when they died, as so many of them did. The constant contact with cancer victims made her increasingly afraid that she might have cancer herself. She was haunted by the idea that any bodily sensation, no matter how innocuous-seeming, could actually be the first sign of a cancer. One of her patients, for example, had learned she had acute leukemia quite by accident when she went to donate blood during a local blood drive. "Anything, a cut that won't heal, a dry cough, a big black and blue mark, could be the first sign," she noted. It seemed as if there was only one brief opportunity to catch a cancer in time, and after that it was too late. As she said, "It seems like the diagnosis is always missed initially, and after that, well, it's just too late." She began checking herself over often, and in examining her breasts one evening, she thought she discovered a mass. Her physician, however, carefully examined her and could find nothing abnormal. Her anxiety had led her to sense a lump when none was there.

This woman was not a hypochondriac, but her work with the sick had caused her to become anxious about her health and thus symptomatic. While her environment was hardly typical, our everyday world has something in common with that cancer ward, and this woman's reactions are like those of many of the worried well who consult physicians. We feel that any ambiguous symptom may be the first sign of a fatal disease, and that you can't take any real reassurance from a normal checkup. We amplify even the most minor symptoms because the possibility of a serious illness is never far from our minds.

Threatened by a Dangerous Environment

The world seems generally filled with peril, jammed with other health hazards in addition to disease. Daily life is a minefield through which we must thread our way: we are in danger of being murdered with a handgun or struck by a drunk driver; there are poisoned Halloween candies and other barely imaginable forms of terrorism; airplane crashes and midair near misses; there are ticks with Lyme disease, mosquitos with AIDS, and "killer" bees. Russell Baker assisted us by gathering in one place "the 125 most publicized things that could get you, listed in alphabetical order," including "a broken ladder rung, casual sex, fiber shortage, a fire ant invasion, icy highway patch, mercury-tainted fish, plaque, poor posture, slippery bathtub, and unvented garage."[12]

Nothing in our environment can be trusted, no matter how comfortable or familiar. Plain old tap water turns out to be a stealthy conveyor of salt, rust, sediment, and toxic substances: contaminants, chemicals, chlorine. If that doesn't do you in, the weather may: the TV weatherman introduces his broadcast with "This heat wave can kill you—the weather today is lethal." Sunlight is another foe because it "weakens" your hair, causes skin cancer, and hastens the signs of aging. And the products we buy every day are booby traps: one car or another is always being recalled just before some critical part gives way; toy manufacturers warn us that our children might get various body parts caught in their products or disassemble them and choke on the parts. The threats come in every conceivable form, from cyanide-laced medicines in the drugstore to food additives in the markets, from nuclear radiation to microwave radiation, from the light of a fluorescent clockface to that of a video display terminal.

We are now much more attuned to the dangers of the workplace, such as asbestos exposure in factories and contact with organic solvents by chemical workers. Even office workers can't escape occupational hazards: "experts" point out that lack of privacy and uncomfortable furniture adversely affect psychological well-being. Going out and having a good time is no solution, because our avocations are as dangerous as our vocations. Swimming might seem fairly safe as long as one is prudent. But as spring arrives, radio spots begin their cautionary drumbeat: "Summer is here and it's the season for swimmer's ear, a condition so painful it can literally make grown men and women cry"; "Running up to the swimming pool before you dive in is a path that can lead to disaster"; et cetera, et cetera, et cetera.

There are, of course, very real reasons to be frightened, including a rising tide of serious environmental health hazards. The litany of toxic chemicals constantly expands, with strange names and acronyms such as dioxin, Mirex, Kepone, and PCB, along with our old favorites, such as lead, mercury, and arsenic, which are still around as well. The skies are tinted with pollution, and low-level radiation leaks from nuclear power plants and from the radioisotopes in commercial waste products. Carcinogens are so widespread that they have been found in the snow of Antarctica and in breast milk; we swallow them with our food and water, inhale them with every breath, and absorb them through our skin.

An entirely new category of hazard is emerging: natural dangers that have always been around us, but that we only just now have recognized. The hazard is not new, but our knowledge of it is. Radon gas is a good example, as are the natural carcinogens found in food; metals such as aluminum and copper; and minerals such as quartz and sand.

Our food is a source of particular concern. The dangers of herbicides and pesticides and food additives (such as food colors and nitrates) have been widely publicized, and many of us try to avoid them. But toxins and carcinogens turn out to be an inextricable part of the food chain, and our dietary intake of natural sources of these substances is many times greater than our intake of the man-made varieties.[13] Of course it is appropriate to eliminate as many of these compounds as possible from our diet, and it is reassuring to know that our food additives are more closely scrutinized and safer than they were at the turn of the century. But our food has not suddenly become a lethal weapon pointed at us. Toxins lie all around us, and always have. They are found in the most delicious and the most familiar foods, such as strawberries, peaches, tea and coffee, onions, and wheat. We have always ingested carcinogens with every meal, and no diet will ever be free of them. What is new is not so much the hazards themselves, but our awareness of them and our fear of them, the sense of being in jeopardy, and at risk within a menacing environment.

A Sense of Bodily Vulnerability

As our environment seems increasingly dangerous, so the human body seems correspondingly fragile. Along with feelings of anxiety and apprehension comes a feeling of physical vulnerability. We don't experience ourselves as rugged and durable, as hardy and naturally resistant to disease, but instead as perpetually on the verge of a breakdown and about to wear out at any moment. The body seems like a dormant adversary, programmed to betray us. Rather than a marvel of reliability, the human heart feels more like a time bomb in our chests, ticking down the minutes to a heart attack. To quote Lewis Thomas again, "The new consensus is that we are badly designed, intrinsically fallible, vulnerable to a host of hostile influences inside and around us, and only precariously alive. We live in danger of falling apart at any moment, and are therefore always in need of surveillance and propping up. Without the professional attention of a health care system, we would fall in our tracks."[14] We overlook the reality that most of us are healthy most of the time, the reality that the human organism has remarkable self-healing abilities and capacities for adaptation and survival.

We are also dissatisfied with our bodies. In nationwide surveys, a surprising 96 percent of Americans say they would like to change something about their bodies. Women are more dissatisfied than men. Seventy-eight percent of women would like to change their weight, 37 percent want to alter their teeth, and 34 percent would change their legs if they could. Among men, 56 percent would change their weight, 39 percent would like to develop their muscles, and 36 percent would like to change their hair if they could.[15] The unease with body weight is especially pervasive. Although only 12 percent of college women were objectively overweight in one study, a full 40 percent of them felt that they were.[16] Looking more generally at all adults, the findings are similar: a much higher proportion of men and women consider themselves obese than actually are.

The prominent narcissistic trends in contemporary American culture, described by Christopher Lasch in *The Culture of Narcissism,* contribute to this collective sense of bodily unease and vulnerability. Lasch describes an element of egotism and self-centeredness, a preoccupation with exterior image and outward appearance and superficial impression, that is evident in our politics, literature, and theater, in business, and in the ascendancy of public relations and advertising.[17] He particularly emphasizes our dedication to the fulfillment of the self. In the past, he argues, Americans devoted themselves to religious salvation, heroic, rugged individualism, or the accumulation of private, family wealth. But in our era, rather than subordinating ourselves to some larger tradition, dedicating ourselves to a cause or to others, we now seek to satisfy our own immediate self-interest, to gratify our unfulfilled desires and impulses without delay.[18] The highest purpose in life is the cultivation of feelings of personal well-being and of physical and psychic health.[19] In the past ten to fifteen years, "being good to yourself" and "feeling good about yourself" have become popular adages; self-absorption has become laudable. One's paramount obligation is to make oneself into as perfect and fulfilled an individual as possible. As a popular song proclaims, "learning to love yourself is the greatest love of all."

The narcissistic character of our epoch is perfectly expressed in the enormous value we place on physique and physical beauty and bodily performance. Our bodies are the most important and precious assets we have, so we strive to care for them and regard them with a mixture of worship, reverence, and adoration that can only be termed narcissistic. Learning about our anatomy and physiology, having cosmetic surgery, vacationing at health resorts, throwing ourselves into Nautilus workouts and triathlons have all become sacred acts of devotion.

Cultural narcissism also fuels the sense of somatic vulnerability and fragility. As we saw in chapter 4, the psychology of narcissism is such that unease and insecurity about ourselves as individuals manifest themselves in feelings of unease and insecurity about our bodies. The fact that our culture displays so many narcissistic features means that deep down, psychologically we tend to feel inadequate, devitalized, deficient, and weak as individuals. Feeling this way about ourselves as people, we begin to feel it about our bodies, and so they seem rickety, flimsy, defective, and unstable. This makes us feel more susceptible to disease and vulnerable to injury. Our sense of bodily and psychic vulnerability is yet another reason why every danger is taken so seriously, every minor symptom seems so threatening, why a healthy checkup fails to reassure.

Cultural narcissism makes even trivial physical imperfections seem shameful. We become uncomfortable with the aging body or the unattractive body, the malodorous body or the imperfect body. So we flock to tanning parlors, scrub with tooth whiteners, buy different deodorants for everything from feet to genitals to underarms to mouth, trying to repair the surface because we feel defective inside.

Our Unease About Aging

One dimension of the climate of dis-ease is a dread of bodily decline. The physical signs and sounds of aging seem horrifying and degrading: the wrinkled skin, thinning hair, and loss of muscle tone; the shuffling gait, snoring, and rumbling stomach. Our dismay about the changes of aging is widespread: in a nationwide poll, one-half (48 percent) of women and one-quarter (27 percent) of men said they wanted to find a way to cover up the evidence of their aging.[20] At the first humiliating evidence of aging that is visible in the mirror, we launch a campaign to camouflage it with plastic surgery, bivouacs at health spas, and renewed resolutions to work out more often. Medical care is supposed to treat old age itself, healthy behavior and an "active lifestyle" to slow the biological clock. When the awkward necessity for bifocal eyeglasses can no longer be denied, for instance, we are urged to buy a pair that "look like regular glasses, because there's no . . . telltale bifocal line . . . to give away the wearer's age."[21] Time's advance must be defied at every turn, since it seems to deplete vigor and vitality and gradually enfeeble us if we let it. One of the worst aspects of the passage of time is that it erodes physical attractiveness. As plastic surgeon Thomas J. Baker put it, "Little lines become creases, creases become crevasses, and crevasses become canyons."[22] So we reach for creams to conceal "unsightly age spots," lest others notice them and care about us less.

D. H. Fisher, in his book *Growing Old in America,* describes how this attitude toward aging has grown over the last two centuries.[23] There was a revolution in attitudes toward the elderly in the United States between 1770 and 1820. The authority of the elderly was undermined, and instead of veneration, the elderly began to be regarded with fear and disapproval. A policy of compulsory retirement was first instituted then, and inheritance law was changed to eliminate the special privileges of eldest children. Census data show that during this period people first began to exaggerate their age downward rather than pretending they were older than they really were, as they had done previously. It became fashionable to look more youthful, and so people stopped powdering their hair to make it white, for example, and started tinting it so as to look younger.

A bona fide cult of youth began late in the nineteenth century and grew rapidly in the twentieth. In the early 1900s, for example, the appearance of older women began to be considered markedly unattractive, inspiring the systematic pursuit of a more youthful appearance through the use of cosmetics and so forth.[24] In the 1960s our adulation of youth reached its apogee, as mature adults mimicked the clothing, language, and the "look" of their adolescent children. Since that time, a pronounced youth-orientation persists, particularly in our emphasis upon physical strength, athletic performance, and youthful appearance. Old age remains a state of having been passed over, of uselessness, rather than of status, respect, and moral authority.[25]

Earlier, we pointed out the paradox that during the current period of collective good health, we have come to feel less healthy—more symptomatic and disabled. Here we see a similar contradiction: during a period of greatly expanded life expectancy, we have come to feel old at an earlier age. We wish more and more for eternal youth, and the years that many other cultures consider to be the prime of life are considered by us to be old age. "Before we're out of our twenties, we begin to feel that as each year passes, we've lost a little something," notes the *Ladies Home Journal*.[26] While still in our thirties, the "midlife" crisis is upon us, signifying that old age looms just around the corner. One's fortieth birthday is experienced as the beginning of the end, the passing from the prime of life,[27] though life is actually only half over. It is not surprising that the age of women coming to plastic surgeons for facelifts is declining: whereas previously such women were usually in their fifties, greater numbers of women in their forties are now having the procedure performed.[28]

Though the story of Ponce de Leon may be more apocryphal than true, it still contains a moral for us. In his fifties, he heard about a spring whose magic waters could reverse the passage of time and restore youth. In 1512 he set out for Bimini, the supposed location of the fountain, but found nothing. Eight years later, now convinced it was in Florida, he set off again, and this time he was killed by an Indian arrow during his fruitless quest. He squandered precious years, and ultimately died, in a vain search for the nonexistent Fountain of Youth.

The fear of aging has left us profoundly uneasy with the passage of time. So we deny the evidence of aging, to ourselves and to others. Rather than gradually relinquishing youth, we fight off the effects of time and cling to the illusion of youth until it is simply no longer tenable. And at this moment of surrender, we become despondent. Yet, as D. H. Fisher writes, "in the end, the discovery that one is old is inescapable."[29] And this discovery is most awful for those who were horrified by its prospect. Our attitude toward age, he concludes, "begins as a loathing of something in others; it ends as loathing of something in oneself. . . . In the end, the cult of youth consumes all of its believers."[30]

Our Aversion to Risk

Our growing dis-ease about health, our sense of environmental menace, our anxiety about the durability of the human body, and our experience of aging go hand in hand with a growing intolerance of all physical hazards and dangers. Almost any risk of harm seems unbearable, whether it be the possibility of an untoward surgical outcome, a drug side effect, a dangerous consumer product, an occupational hazard, or a collapsing highway bridge. We are in a perpetual state of alarm about the daily health risks we run, the dangers inherent in everything we do, from changing a light bulb to mowing the lawn. Since all risks must be eliminated, we have to learn how to shovel snow without precipitating a heart attack, how to go to the beach without succumbing to heat stroke or sunburn, and how to carry golf clubs without causing low-back strain.

Once disease and suffering are no longer fatalistically accepted as phenomena over which man has no control, an entire range of misfortunes and mishaps becomes progressively harder to bear, and the risk of incurring them seems insupportable.[31] Thus we are obsessed not just with minimizing physical risk, but with eliminating it. No risk, no hazard, is acceptable, even if it is extremely small. The "act of God," the unforeseeable mishap, the uncertain outcome have all become intolerable. If anything goes wrong and results in injury or death, an error must have been made and someone must be at fault. When the U.S. Weather Bureau is *successfully* sued for failing to predict an ocean storm that killed several fishermen, we are trying to deny that there are uncontrollable factors in going to sea, that it is an inherently risky business. The courts, legislatures, and special-interest groups contend that no price is too great to pay in order to remove a source of physical jeopardy.

Even the long-shot odds of contracting a very rare disease become something we try to eliminate. Thus the formation of the National Organization for Rare Disorders, which solicits contributions with the admonition "Someone you know has a rare disorder. That may be fatal or disabling. That many doctors don't recognize." Part of the problem here is that because our anxiety is so great, it has become easy to confuse relative risks with absolute risks. Relative risk (for example, the increased likelihood of your getting a certain cancer if you drink coffee) is important for statistical research and for the study of large populations, but it has little to do with the actual chances that you will come down with that cancer. That is a function of absolute risk, the actual frequency of the disorder in the population. If the cancer we are talking about is a rare one, and your risk of developing it is 1 in 100,000, say, then even if coffee drinking triples your risk, your chance is now still only 3 in 100,000, a slim chance either way. But at present we feel so generally unsafe that we are afraid of many quite unlikely events.

Our risk aversion is manifested in an intolerance of medical uncertainty, whether in medical practice or in medical research.[32] It is also apparent in our unforgiving reactions to accidental injury and in the high costs we pay to avoid some dangers in the workplace.

Twenty years ago, when a physician delivered a baby who turned out to be less than perfect, the development was considered an act of God. "Today, there are no more acts of God," an obstetrician observes. No matter what happens, "parents feel that you should have been able to do something."[33] Medical malpractice claims have tripled in the last ten years and plaintiffs are winning record settlements. Has the quality of medical care deteriorated that catastrophically? Are there that many more untoward outcomes than there were ten years ago? No. Behind the mushrooming medical malpractice actions lies the fantasy that nothing should ever go wrong in the medical-care process and the belief that it is possible to prevent all adverse results. A Boston attorney active in the malpractice field notes, "The question of who is likely to be sued does not revolve around who is . . . negligent as much as who fails to meet the expectations of patients."[34] In many malpractice verdicts, we hold physicians liable for the scientific limitations and human uncertainties that are inherent in clinical medicine.

Patients and their families tend to think of medical care as an exact science. But despite its technological trappings, medicine is still a matter of probabilities, estimates, and even unknowns. It remains more art and judgment, inference and guesswork, than certainty and science. Deciding which drug to prescribe is not as simple as looking it up in the *Physician's Desk Reference*. Medical outcomes are neither always foreseeable nor always favorable. A weakened and undernourished eighty-three-year-old woman with leukemia nonetheless bounces back from a massive heart attack to leave the hospital eight days later, while a healthy young father admitted for elective surgery on a small hernia develops blood-pressure problems during the operation and dies.

Even with the best medical care, the outcome is not always happy. All drugs have adverse side effects, whether we like it or not; if they are used enough times in enough patients, someone is eventually going to be harmed by every one of them. Physicians are fallible and make errors in judgment, as appalling as that sounds; if enough physicians make enough decisions, eventually someone will make an incorrect one. That is not a law of medicine, it is a law of probability. Laboratory equipment malfunctions, medical records are misplaced, surgical incisions become infected. But we are so afraid of illness and injury, so anxious about our health and safety, that we deny the very idea that things go wrong, that fallibility exists, that mistakes and mishaps and bad luck are a part of medicine.

Our risk aversion is so intense that at times we run blindly away from a trivial threat only to fall headlong into the arms of a serious one. Whooping cough, a major killer of children until the 1940s, was largely eradicated with public inoculation programs using the DPT vaccine. Now the incidence of whooping cough is rising again, and health officials are concerned about increasing numbers of parents who refuse to inoculate their children because of the rare instances in which the vaccine has resulted in permanent brain damage. But the fact is that the chances of being harmed by whooping cough are ten times greater than those of being harmed by the vaccine. Likewise, the epidemic of liability lawsuits against drug and medical-equipment manufacturers has on occasion had undesirable consequences. As a result of the legal climate, one of the better intrauterine birth-control devices has been taken off the market, and several important pieces of medical equipment are no longer being manufactured. The makers of vaccines have been particularly hard hit by lawsuits, which in one instance have increased the price of a single immunization from 45¢ to $11.40 in only four years.[35]

This same intolerance of medical risk is apparent in our attitudes toward medical research. Thus we ask that there be no danger in recombinant DNA research, as if medical research could be devoid of untoward consequences. While extensive, rigorous evaluation of new drugs is absolutely necessary before they can be approved for clinical use, there have been instances in which the introduction of useful drugs has been delayed because of excessive fears about infrequent adverse reactions and unlikely side effects. Even in the treatment of the terminally ill, where one might expect greater tolerance of long-term risks, the introduction of effective agents is sometimes delayed excessively.[36] The current climate is such that even a single death attributed to a useful drug generates sensational adverse publicity, can cost tens of millions of dollars in lawsuits, and can cause the drug to be taken off the market.

Our aversion to the risk of injury is also apparent in our attitudes toward consumer-product safety and liability. While there are many egregious examples of manufacturer liability, some lawsuits and court decisions reflect the underlying premise that accidents and injuries simply should never happen. If they do, then by definition a mistake has been made and someone is at fault. So now you can't assemble a folding chair or unpack a toaster without wending your way through a thicket of tags, stickers, and booklets warning against every imaginable misuse. Product designers and manufacturers are held responsible for even the most improbable adverse outcomes, as if every possible malfunction of the product could and should have been anticipated. When a sixteen-month-old child choked on a peanut butter sandwich, the family sued the peanut butter manufacturer, claiming that there should have been a warning on the jar that peanut butter could be dangerous. (The case was settled out of court.) While such a suit sounds farfetched, there have been many others like it, some of them even successful.[37] The mere fact that such extreme legal actions occur at all indicates how far our obsession with safety has gone.

Abhorrence of risk is similarly reflected in some of our occupational safety and health standards. The development of these standards was a major public-health advance, one that has clearly made the workplace far safer today than it was. But recently we have promulgated some standards that are extremely costly to comply with and are aimed at reducing the likelihood of diseases and injuries that are already extremely rare.[38] These standards may still be completely justified; the point is only that we have at times been willing to go to very great lengths to protect ourselves against some very unlikely events. The elimination of all left turns would lower the number of traffic accidents, but does that mean we should outlaw them?

The more we believe that disease can be controlled and avoided, the more intolerant we become of a wider array of physical hazards and dangers. In our extreme risk aversion, the harsh reality we try to ignore is that some risk is simply inherent in life—that living itself is "hazardous to your health." We are in jeopardy crossing the street, taking a bath, or living near an airport. There are, and always will be, injurious events that we cannot anticipate, and not every such mishap has a culprit.

Feeling Besieged

Good health is experienced as a tenuous state that requires our constant attention and effort. Behind the hazards posed by disease and aging, we glimpse rank upon rank of other mortal threats—injury, accident, contamination, contagion, pollution, assault—which make life all the more dangerous and unsafe. We feel defenseless and vulnerable in the face of so many corporeal hazards and sources of harm. It is a feeling of being under siege.

This siege mentality is perfectly expressed in some of our attitudes toward the AIDS epidemic. While AIDS is undeniably a major public-health threat, a lethal epidemic of historic proportions, nonetheless, we can see in our reactions to it some expressions of excessive panic. AIDS, as prevalent and as deadly as it is, is only transmitted by intimate sexual contact, transfusions of blood containing the virus, the use of contaminated hypodermic needles, or from mother to fetus. The risk of contagion by casual contact is considered negligible. Yet 47 percent of people think that AIDS can be contracted from a drinking glass, and 28 percent believe it can be picked up from a toilet seat.[39] Drastic measures, such as the quarantine of people who could unknowingly spread the virus, such as food handlers, barbers, doctors, and nurses (as well as, of course, AIDS patients themselves), have been advocated. The terror of AIDS is so overwhelming that attempts at mass education just seem to create more fear and confusion. After blood banks requested that members of high-risk groups refrain from donating blood, 26 percent of the respondents in a Roper poll expressed the belief that they could *acquire* AIDS by donating blood.

Our terror of AIDS is similar to people's responses to the plagues and epidemics of the past, but then we knew far less about how these diseases were transmitted. Lance Morrow, writing in *Time* magazine about the epidemic of yellow fever in Philadelphia in 1793, captures perfectly today's atmosphere and its atavistic quality: "A plague mentality set in. Friends recoiled from one another. If they met by chance, they did not shake hands but nodded distantly and hurried on. The very air felt diseased. People dodged to the windward of those they passed. They sealed themselves in their houses. . . . Many adopted a policy of savage self-preservation, all sentiment heaved overboard like ballast. Husbands deserted stricken wives, parents abandoned children. The corpses of even the wealthy were carted off unattended, to be shoveled under without ceremony or prayer. . . . [In] the plague mentality death drifts through human blood or saliva. It commutes by bugbite or kiss or who knows what. It travels in mysterious ways, and everything, everyone, becomes suspect: a toilet seat, a child's cut, an act of love. . . . People . . . peer intently at one another as if to detect the telltale change, the secret lesion, the sign that someone has crossed over, is not himself anymore, but one of *them,* alien and lethal. . . . But, like a plague itself, a plague mentality seems an anachronism in the elaborately doctored postindustrial U.S. . . . AIDS, implacable and thus far incurable, comes as a shock. It arrives like a cannibal at the picnic and calmly starts eating the children."[40]

We react to feeling besieged by trying to fortify ourselves, to become as self-sufficient, totally fit, and physically invulnerable as possible. The commercial health and wellness industry promotes this sense of emergency and impending crisis. Self-help books are regarded as lifesaving. The notions of preventive medicine and health promotion also foster this state-of-emergency mentality by implying that survival depends upon constant vigilance and a regular sequence of examinations. Thus healthy people start storing up their own blood in commercial blood banks, stockpiling it for a rainy day, so it will be there in the event that they need a blood transfusion in the future. "Why take chances . . . Start storing *your own* blood today. Collecting, freezing and safely storing units of your own blood for your own use is a medical procedure whose time has come," says the advertisement.

The image of stockpiling one's own blood for an approaching medical Armageddon characterizes the contemporary experience. At any moment you may be stricken or wounded and require a blood transfusion to save your life. You must anticipate this and prepare for it now by taking out a new kind of health insurance: not by putting money in the bank, but by putting blood in the bank. Contrast this with the bomb-shelter craze of the 1950s and 1960s. Even more dangerous now than the Russians is the danger of disease. If there are still people out there building bomb shelters, they are surely health conscious enough to be including several units of their own blood and a copy of the *Royal Canadian Air Force Fitness Manual* along with their freeze-dried foods and radiation detectors.

The image of one's own personal blood bank embodies another aspect of the present climate. It is not just being sick and requiring a blood transfusion that we fear; it is also needing someone else when we are sick. We can't rely upon anyone for a lifesaving gift of blood, because they might give us AIDS or hepatitis (or both) along with it. A hand extended in assistance could prove fatal. As the advertisement says, "Your own blood is the safest to receive. There is no risk of exposure to infectious disease from transfusion of another person's blood." So not only do we face a perilous future, but we face it with a lessened sense of community, wary of the need to depend on others, without mutual support and aid.

Survivalism:
It's Time to Circle the Wagons

When it feels as if we are living in a state of siege, and life is reduced to an obstacle course, then sheer survival—simply making it through the course—becomes the paramount concern.[41] It is time to draw the wagons into a circle, to "cut out the fat," to "tighten our belts." Confronted with a threatening and hazardous world, we try to assert control in the one sphere of influence we believe is left to us: our bodies and our personal behavior. As one respondent to a *Psychology Today* survey put it: "Health is the only thing left in my life that I can control."[42]

Survival is on our minds since it feels as if disaster is looming just over the horizon. It's time to make certain we can look after our own medical needs by stocking up on medical encyclopedias and learning to do cardiopulmonary resuscitation and the Heimlich maneuver. Just to be sure, why not double-check that everything in the medicine cabinet came with tamper-proof seals. And it is a good idea to get a Medic-Alert bracelet and write out a living will, because who knows when the end might come. We could try to bolster our immunity with a new diet, because it's hard not to worry about the specter of AIDS, even when we're not in a high-risk group. And don't forget to get a flu shot.

The impetus toward maintaining personal safety and personal control is intensified when life is experienced as insecure and uncertain, when it seems to be filled with lethal threats that are remote, difficult to measure, and hard to combat. People do whatever they can as individuals to maximize their health and their chances of survival, to make their personal world feel safer, to keep themselves out of harm's way. So we install fire alarms, "buckle up for safety," buy flood and earthquake insurance, install a water purifier on the kitchen faucet, and acquire a handgun.

This interest in survival can be seen in marathon running and other extreme forms of exercise, where we flirt with mortality in the context of sports. The marathon is an unusual sport in that, for most entrants, the point is not to win but merely to finish.[43] The objective of the race is to survive it. Even the losers in marathons are heroes, as epitomized by the young woman who received a standing ovation as she crawled to the finish line in the 1984 Olympics.[44] In triathlons, "iron man" contests, and other such events, the objective is simply to endure the rigors of the event. A radical example is the Western States Endurance Run, which begins in Squaw Valley, California, and extends over 100 miles of wild and rough terrain. The course climbs 17,000 feet, through temperatures from just above freezing to over 100 degrees. Runners must contend with snow, mud, and rattlesnakes. *Ultrasport* magazine notes, "The race has a fine tradition: No one has died."[45] *Outside* magazine describes it as "the hardest, sickest, ultra-endurance event of them all . . . a day of living death."[46]

Much of what we are doing is beneficial, or at the least is not harmful. But it is important to note that with it we are only treating a symptom—our feeling of being besieged—and not the underlying cause of the symptom—the things that besiege us. And herein lies a danger. As Lewis Thomas has written, "Our preoccupation with personal health may be a symptom of copping out, an excuse for running upstairs to recline on a couch, sniffing the air for contaminants, spraying the room with deodorants, while just outside, the whole of society is coming undone."[47] Faced with a world whose dangers seem out of control, each of us retreats to shore up his own physical integrity, to attempt to ensure his survival by building his resistance and stretching his endurance. Powerless to stem the seepage of toxic wastes, unable to stuff the looming nuclear genie back into the bottle, at the mercy of some psychopath who would assault us on the street, we switch to bottled water, fortify our diet, head for the basement to work out. To the most pessimistic of observers, some of this frantic health promotion has the disquieting aura of rearranging deck chairs on the *Titanic*.

A Nation of Worried Well

We must be careful not to become a nation of worried well. The possibility of physical danger seems to lurk everywhere, hovering over everything we do, not only in the form of disease, but of accident, injury, and aging as well. We're always in jeopardy, afraid for ourselves and our futures, for our children, even for our pets. Our bodies are never fit enough or immune enough or strong enough. Life seems far too risky, and even something as predictable as the passage of time seems enervating and vitiating.

In earlier chapters, we examined four characteristics of our contemporary culture: a heightened health consciousness, which focuses our *attention* on health matters; a medicalization of society, which supplies the *context* for our experience of illness; an ideology of control over health, which provides a *belief* system about our bodily sensations; and a *mood* of dis-ease, which colors our experience of physical well-being and security. These four cultural characteristics amplify personal feelings of ill health. They also supply us with a vocabulary for expressing our health concerns and with ways of acting them out. Personal health concerns, even of a hypochondriacal nature, can now be discussed in a socially acceptable language: "modifying risk factors," attaining a state of "wellness," "getting into shape," "doing something good for your body," and the rest. And we can act out our concerns in socially sanctioned and even fashionable ways, from dosing ourselves with nutritional supplements, to self-diagnosis at home with do-it-yourself kits, to cataloging our skin moles and our sleep habits.

Why are we so worried? To start with, predisposing risk factors are so widely appreciated, and diagnostic technology so powerful and so discerning, that a state of apparent good health seems no more than a screen for troubles hidden and troubles to come. It has become harder to trust one's intuitive feeling of good health and to take comfort in the fact that we have no symptoms. It is also more difficult for healthy people to experience a feeling of well-being because we have been so inculcated with the seeming necessity of maintaining a constant vigil over the state of our bodies. Moreover, the cultural atmosphere of anxiety makes good health seem tenuous and precarious, and makes life seem like a hazardous patrol through enemy territory.

Once we do note a symptom or a sign, we have been indoctrinated into appraising it in the worst possible light—as something worthy of careful evaluation and immediate attention, something disabling and disruptive. Any sensation, no matter how common, no matter how innocuous, could be the harbinger of some lethal condition or other. Even the undiagnosable aches and pains that we have long endured deserve careful scrutiny because they might now be recognizable as signs of some new disease that has just been discovered. In addition, the climate of dis-ease amplifies symptoms, making them more noxious, more disturbing, and more threatening.

Once you actually fall ill, you take on an enormously expanded role: being a patient is now far more demanding and more exacting than it was. You acquire more factual information about your illness, learn to manage it, and observe and regard yourself in a clinical fashion. To the burdens and fears of being ill have been added the responsibilities and duties of being your own physician. And you not only have the responsibility for recuperation, but even (by implication) for the course and outcome of your illness. Illness is more frightful and coping with it is more difficult now because the religious side of medicine, the extended family, and the social support systems that once would have helped you bear and cope with it are in decline today. The atmosphere of dis-ease affects both our experience of illness and our understanding of disease. The illness experience is made to seem more worrisome and more perilous, and the disease that afflicts us seems more grave and more menacing.

Finally, as a result of all these societal changes, the outcome of your illness, if it is anything short of total recovery, is more likely to leave you disappointed. The heightened health consciousness and the climate of dis-ease make disability and frailty and infirmity seem intolerable. Medicalization has led us to believe that almost everything should be cured, if not through the wonders of biomedicine, then through our own efforts. Our belief in our control of disease leaves us feeling more disappointed and angry and personally responsible when the outcome is less than ideal.

CHAPTER 9

The Paradox of Health

"He Who Lives Medically Lives Miserably"

SENECA, THE ROMAN SCHOLAR AND THINKER, observed 2,000 years ago: "No man can have a peaceful life who thinks too much about lengthening it." He could have been speaking to us. Despite enormous improvements in health status, we are not confident of our physical well-being. Our highly successful crusade against disease has paradoxically resulted in dis-ease. Having painstakingly forged taut, muscular bodies, we still don't feel rugged, robust, and secure. Plagued by the seeming necessity of constant medical attention, we can't live exuberantly but instead feel timid and apprehensive about our health. Our medical efforts have by some perverse trick of fate left us with diminished, rather than enhanced, feelings of well-being. There is a paradox: the healthier we become, the more concerned with health we become. And yet real health encompasses a sense of physical well-being, of vitality and hardiness, as surely as it does the absence of disease.

A Latin proverb says it: "He who lives medically lives miserably." The more assiduously we exercise and go for checkups, the more a feeling of genuine healthiness eludes us. The more carefully we scrutinize ourselves for ailments, the more things we find wrong with us. The more we diet, the more frustrated we become with our flab. Though we live longer, we feel old sooner. The more undesirable states we medicalize, the more diseases there are to suffer from. The more we equate health with total well-being, the more pervasive illness becomes. We extend the boundaries of patienthood so much that more of us live more of our lives in that territory. It is a vicious cycle.

The feeling of physical well-being is elusive in the same way that happiness is; it is more a by-product of successful living than it is an objective that can be attained by striving for it directly. You can't *make* yourself happy, just as you can't *make* yourself fall asleep or relax or remember a name; rather, you can only *allow* these things to occur. The feeling of physical well-being seems to be similar. The pursuit of healthiness is a peculiar process in which the harder we try to hit the bull's-eye, the more likely we are to miss the mark.

Like a dog chasing its tail, our attempts to pacify our concerns themselves generate new concerns. For health reasons, we pass up sugar for saccharin, but then questions are raised about the safety of saccharin, so we switch to cyclamate; cyclamate is banned because of a suspected link to cancer, so we use aspartame; then aspartame is suspected of causing seizures; finally, in 1986, the Food and Drug Administration concludes that sugar consumption does *not* significantly affect the development of diabetes, high blood pressure, heart disease, or behavioral problems. We have come full circle. There are other, similar scenarios: we switch to decaffeinated coffee, only to worry about the danger of the decaffeination process; we substitute fish for meat, only to discover mercury in the fish. First we treat our illnesses with more and more pills, and then we worry about the nutritional value of the medications, so that pills themselves are now promoted as sodium-free or calcium-rich or caffeine-free. Either they constitute such a large part of our diet that they really are an important source of nutrition, or we are preoccupied with something inconsequential.

The pervasive feeling of dis-ease in an age of vastly improved health is possible because the relationship between actual health and perceived health is so surprisingly fickle, as we have seen. Smoothly functioning organs don't guarantee a feeling of vitality or healthiness. This lack of one-to-one correspondence between objective and subjective health reaches its acme in the peculiarly modern state of being objectively almost normal and yet subjectively dead at the same time. This occurs in people who are comatose and terminally ill, but who are kept "alive" with life-support systems. The patient's physiological functions have all been normalized with the most sophisticated medical technology, while as a meaningful entity—a person—he has long since ceased to exist. He thus symbolizes both the omnipotence and the impotence of modern medicine. (This grotesque situation has sometimes been referred to at the hospital where I work as "dying the Harvard way.") In the black humor of high-tech medicine, the patient is then finally transferred from the intensive-care unit to the "eternal-care unit." (This ironic argot, though seemingly callous, at least seems preferable to that used by public-relations officials who announced the death of a celebrity patient by saying, "The patient did not fulfill his wellness potential.")

Prisoners of Health

People today do not feel healthier than in the past. Quite to the contrary: in national polls, the proportion of respondents who are satisfied with their health and physical condition has dropped from 61 percent in the 1970s to 55 percent in the mid-1980s.[1]

Survey data show that we are more bothered by trivial symptoms and more disabled by minor ailments than we once were. In large-scale, community-wide surveys conducted in the 1920s, the average American reported 0.82 episodes of serious, acute illness per year. But when the same information was sought from Americans in the early 1980s, the average person reported 2.12 serious, acute illnesses per year.*[2] Thus people now consider themselves to have two and one-half times more acute illnesses than they did fifty years ago, despite the passage of a half-century in which their collective health has actually improved dramatically and in which antibiotics were introduced for the treatment of acute infections. In addition, people now report that these illness episodes last longer than those reported in the late 1920s. Then, people reported that their "disabling" illness episodes lasted an average of sixteen days, while today that same disabling episode lasts nineteen days.[3]

There are several possible explanations for these reports of more frequent and more prolonged acute illnesses nowadays, since interpreting and comparing these kinds of long-term studies over time is tricky. But the general explanation, which seems to fit the findings best, is that people have developed a lower threshold, and a lower tolerance, for the experience of illness over this period of time. There appears to have been an increase in the standard we use for judging our health, so that we are now more aware of, and more disturbed by, symptoms and impairments that were previously deemed less significant.

The same trend has been documented in studies of the more recent past. Between 1957 and 1976, researchers from the University of Michigan's Institute for Social Research interviewed nationwide samples of 2,500 normal adults. They were asked whether they had experienced symptoms such as shortness of breath, heart palpitations, and pain, and whether they felt healthy enough to work and to do things they would like to do. Both men and women reported more ill health in 1976 than they did in 1957.[4] Also, there was a decline in the number of people who reported having no symptoms. The researchers drew two conclusions about the increase in the experience of ill health over that period: first,

---

* "Serious, acute illnesses" are defined in these surveys as any disorder that disabled the person for at least one day, or that required medical attention, but that lasted fewer than three months. Chronic illnesses, therefore, are not included.

that people have become more inclined to notice these bodily experiences and consider them to be symptoms of illness; and second, that there are now fewer constraints on admitting that we are sick and reporting this to an interviewer—i.e., there is a greater readiness to acknowledge that we feel ill than there used to be.

The trend toward experiencing longer disability episodes has also been seen in recent studies of men and women aged forty-five and older. These studies confirm that people now experience more reduced-activity days and days in bed, *per condition,* than they did in the 1950s.[5] Apparently, people adopt the sick role more readily than they used to, perhaps in part because disability is more socially sanctioned now. Sick-leave policies, public-assistance programs, and pension plans for the disabled make longer disability more remunerative and more acceptable.[6] Nationwide surveys undertaken for the National Health Survey show that among Americans who were in the work force between 1961 and 1976, there have been increases in the percentage of people reporting health limitations upon their activity, in the number of acute conditions they report, and the number of restricted-activity days per person per year.[7] These data are difficult to interpret, however, since there have also been changes in the labor force during this period.*

A similar tendency has been reported among college students. University health services report increasing numbers of medical excuses for postponing final examinations. These requests for make-up examinations reflect the fact that students are reluctant to take an examination unless they feel they are in top physical condition. This criterion of being in top condition in turn reflects an expanded definition of illness, and the changes that have occurred in the commonly

---

* These changes include a higher proportion of females in the labor force, more extensive health-insurance coverage, and a decline in the average age of the work force.

accepted grounds for exemption from normal role performance.[8]

In studies comparing illness perception among people of different social classes, those of higher social position, who are generally in better health than those of lower social position, report more mild symptoms such as cuts and bruises, skin problems, and upper-respiratory-tract illnesses.[9] This seems to suggest that as you become healthier and have fewer serious illnesses, you notice and focus upon more trivial disturbances. When the inhabitants of poorer nations are compared to people from wealthier countries with a higher health status, both groups describe about the same number of symptoms.[10] That is, the disease-afflicted Indian or Arab doesn't seem to recognize or report more symptoms than the healthier American. Because they are so accustomed to serious disease and disability, the inhabitants of these less healthy societies report fewer symptoms and fewer illneses than Western physicians who examine them expect them to report. Perhaps the total number of physical symptoms that the human being can experience is relatively fixed and fairly constant, regardless of how seriously sick he is, and therefore the healthier American and the sicker Arab have about the same number of complaints.[11] This might partially explain what has been happening over the years in America.

The Biological Paradox:
A Bitter Pill

The awful biological truth is that sickness will always be with us. The absence of disease is incompatible with life; to put it another way, life is the leading cause of death. Though we may conquer individual diseases one by one, the sum total of these separate triumphs will not be the elimination of all disease. New diseases will arise to replace the old. AIDS is an all-too-vivid illustration. Yet, as we have seen, there is a widespread fantasy that the very existence of disease in general is a problem that can be solved through scientific advance and technological expertise, and that the result will be an end to sickness and bodily afflictions. The fact remains, however, that disease is an inextricable part of life itself and cannot be excised or eliminated.

Health and Disease: Two Sides of the Same Coin

A disease-free life is not possible because health and disease are two sides of the same coin. Normality is inconceivable without abnormality. Sickness will always be a fact of human existence, as it is a fact for all living things that evolve over time. Our vegetables and our lawns become diseased, as do our pets and even our vermin.

The state that we call health is actually the successful adaptation of the individual to the demands of his environment. Health and sickness refer to the moment-to-moment success or failure of this adaptation, the adequacy of our response to the challenges and stresses we are constantly subjected to.[12] Health is a temporary state of being, not an enduring characteristic. It is a constantly changing equilibrium between the organism and its environment, a fluid balance, as René Dubos pointed out in *The Mirage of Health*.[13] Since our environment is constantly changing, health can only be a transient state. Sooner or later, there will come an environmental change to which we are unable to adapt. Health cannot be captured and preserved, like knowledge, but instead, like wisdom, is a by-product of successfully coping with the environment.

If your physician pronounces you healthy after a checkup, he is not describing an inherent characteristic of your body, like your height or hair color. Rather, he refers to the successful fit between your body and the environmental demands being made on it at the time. Your good health means that your body has been able to keep its internal temperature constant as you moved from the cold parking lot where you parked your car into your physician's overheated waiting room. It means that your immune system has been able to restrain the viruses you've been exposed to and has kept you from catching a cold. It is to these successful adaptations, and to a thousand others like them, that the term *health* really applies.

In addition to the environmental changes that occur naturally, man constantly manipulates and alters his environment and in so doing introduces new elements that require further adaptation. He builds cities that breed rats and infection. He invents automobiles that pollute the air and accidentally injure him. He experiments with dangerous chemicals and creates pesticides and toxins. Man's environment is not fixed but dynamic; man, therefore, will always face new threats to health and fail to adapt successfully to some. The result will be termed "sickness."

Dying of Old Age Rather Than Disease

There is another biological law that curtails the success of our quest for health: the physical decline of aging. Old age is not a disorder we are about to cure. Medical care cannot lengthen life indefinitely. There is such a thing as a "natural death." Indeed, the length of a human life appears to be relatively fixed. Life span (the maximal age obtainable by a member of a species) is not elastic. Even if we could eliminate all disease, people would still die. They would succumb to old age rather than to disease, but die they would. It has been estimated that in such an ideal world, where no one died prematurely from disease, the average citizen would die of old age somewhere around age eighty-five.[14] Two-thirds of the inhabitants of this disease-free Eden would die between eighty-one and eighty-nine years of age. If right now we were able to eliminate all violent and traumatic deaths, which account for more than half of the premature deaths occurring in those under forty, then, owing to medical advances, our average life expectancy would already begin to approach eighty-five, the theoretical limit to human life.

Several lines of evidence indicate that people would still die of old age even if we were to eliminate disease. First, when we study the age distributions of various societies, we find that the proportion of people who live to extreme old age, say, beyond 100, is quite similar in many different countries and in many different epochs. In England from 1837 to the present, there has been a dramatic increase in the *average* life expectancy, while the proportion of people who live to be 100 has remained the same. The statistics are strikingly similar in most developed societies: about one person in every 10,000 reaches 100. Furthermore, careful examination of people's claims to extreme longevity reveals another consistent finding in many different societies and in many different places: the oldest documented age appears to be between 110 and 114. Despite reports in the popular press, there has not been rigorous documentation of unusual societies that are blessed with exceptional longevity. Careful scientific study seems to show, sad to say, that those mountaintop towns purportedly populated by 115-year-old yogurt-eating Russians are actually populated by 85-year-old yogurt-eating Russians. Thus, in spite of our success in increasing *average* longevity, the *maximum* life span has not changed. As people age they become increasingly illness-prone and, in spite of improved medical care, will eventually die at term, as it were.[15] Medicine cannot turn back the biological clock.

A second line of evidence is experimental. Cells grown outside of the body in tissue culture reproduce themselves only a limited number of times. After a certain number of generations, such cells first fail to grow and then stop dividing altogether, even though they are kept in exactly the same conditions and continue to receive the same nutrients. Each type of cell has a limit to the number of times it can reproduce itself, and the cells belonging to species with longer life spans divide more times in tissue culture before dying out. In short, senescence is programmed into the life of the normal cell. Death is an inextricable part of cellular life and not just the result of disease.

A third line of evidence involves the progressive decline in the functional capacity of the organs of the body throughout adult life. When we are young adults, each of our organs has a built-in biological redundancy, a functional capacity four to ten times greater than that necessary to keep us alive. The liver, for example, can metabolize ten times more of the body's chemical by-products than it is actually called upon to do, and the kidneys are capable of filtering ten times more waste products out of the bloodstream than they have to. But once the individual reaches the age of thirty and begins passing through a *healthy* middle age, the maximal functional capacity of each organ gradually declines. Thus, even without becoming sick, people would eventually die a natural death because their organs would no longer function adequately.

"The Failures of Success"[16]

While in recent years medical care has become more effective and more accessible, and the health practices of the American people have improved, the prevalence of chronic and degenerative disorders has risen. It has been estimated that 80 percent of all disease in our country is now chronic and degenerative, while fifty years ago only 30 percent was.[17] We have, in effect, exchanged acute, life-threatening diseases early in life for chronic, disabling ones later on. Most of the killers that caused sudden and untimely death (such as pneumonia, tuberculosis, and childhood infections) can now be successfully prevented or treated. But the people saved from these untimely deaths now live long enough to be afflicted by diabetes, osteoarthritis, cataracts, and degenerative disorders—the things that come with longevity and that we are less successful at treating. In addition, while we are better at preventing *death* from sudden, life-threatening illnesses, some of the survivors of such illnesses are left with residual disability and even invalidism. For example, your odds of surviving a serious stroke are now better, but you may be left paralyzed and unable to speak. You may now live through a heart attack that would have been fatal in the past, but you may remain disabled by congestive heart failure. Thus, while more effective medical care enables us to live longer, the *proportion* of life spent in ill health has actually *increased.*

Furthermore, people now live longer with their chronic illnesses because while improved medical care doesn't prevent or cure the disorders, it slows their progression and postpones death from them. Chronic-disease sufferers tended in the past to die more often from acute infections superimposed on the chronic disease than from the chronic disease itself. And since we can now cure many of these acute infections, these patients live longer than they used to.[18] The result of this lengthening of lives is an increase in the proportion of the population suffering from the condition. We use the term "the failures of success" to describe the phenomenon whereby some diseases actually become *more, rather than less,* prevalent as a result of medical advances.[19] An example is dementia, whose prevalence is increasing in part because we are better at treating the terminal events (such as pneumonia and kidney failure) that used to kill demented people. To take another example, people with Down's syndrome now often survive into their fifties, and, for the first time in history, we have significant numbers of seventy-year-old mongoloids.[20] The prevalence of mongolism, therefore, is rising.

The aging of our population is also important here. It affects the kinds of diseases we suffer from because older people get different diseases, and more diseases, than younger people do. And the elderly are the most rapidly growing segment of the population. In 1900, only 4 percent of Americans were over sixty-five, and in 1940 less than 7 percent of us had attained this age. But by 1980 the figure had risen to

11.3 percent and by the year 2000 it is predicted that 12.2 percent of Americans will be sixty-five or older.[21] What is most important from our point of view is that an older population means a sicker population. Physical health in general begins to decline after age forty-five, and the incidence of chronic and degenerative illness rises with longevity.

The Paradox of Medical Care
The Limits of Personal Care

We seem to be approaching a point of diminishing returns where increasing amounts of personal medical care do not improve mortality rates very much.[22] Studies of countries with high standards of living and of medical care disclose that further increases in direct expenditures for personal medical care do little to reduce death rates.[23] Mortality rates alone, of course, are really inadequate indicators of health status, because they tell us little about disability, suffering, and the quality of life. And personal medical care may actually have its greatest impact not in increasing longevity, but in making people's lives more functional and more comfortable. But modern biomedicine's inability to lower mortality further is nonetheless important for us to note, since it is one source of dissatisfaction and disillusionment with the growing medicalization of life.*

One reason that medical care has so little impact on mortality is that the most common causes of death today (like alcoholism, lung cancer, automobile accidents, suicide) have prominent behavioral and environmental causes. Progress against them requires alterations in behavior and in the environment (like curtailing the use of alcohol, controlling pol-

---

* This does not address the very real problem of barriers, both financial and circumstantial, that exist in the access to care. While we have very high standards of personal medical care indeed, there are great inequities in the delivery of that care. Large numbers of people in the United States remain underserved and underinsured, and thus do not benefit from the advances of modern biomedicine. Improvements in the delivery of medical care, making it more available to those in need, would still improve our collective health status.

lution, equipping cars with air bags, and a willingness to engage in psychotherapy), not just in personal medical care. Because modern medicine treats diseased organs better than unhealthy lifestyles and environmental influences, it is not surprising that it now has a limited impact on overall death rates.

While we have recently begun to stress the need to modify behavior, historically as a society we have placed greater emphasis on technology-intensive, hospital-based, heroic care for the critically ill. These sorts of medical interventions have a small impact upon the collective health of the whole society, because while they may be effective, the number of people saved by them is a relatively small fraction of the total population. For example, because coronary-care units improve our chances of surviving a serious heart attack, they would seem to be one of modern medicine's most impressive triumphs. But it turns out that although these units are beneficial for some heart-attack victims they don't seem to be very crucial for most such patients.[24] Studies have compared heart-attack patients admitted to hospital coronary-care units with heart-attack patients who were simply treated at home with bed rest. About one-quarter of heart-attack patients were so seriously ill that they were immediately hospitalized and so were not included in these studies. But the remaining 75 percent of patients were randomly admitted to the coronary-care unit or treated at home. Most studies show that these two treatment groups did equally well, at least as far as short-term survival is concerned. Furthermore, the people who are saved by this high-technology medicine often go on to die of another complication or illness relatively soon thereafter; in saving them, we have simply postponed their deaths briefly rather than avoiding them. Thus it appears that infants who are saved in the first month of life by neonatal intensive-care units are still much more likely to die before the end of the first year of life.[25]

By contrast, public-health measures that prevent disease

from occurring in a large population, rather than treating it once it has struck a smaller number of people, tend to have a more significant effect on collective health status.[26] For example, a report by the National Academy of Sciences' Institute of Medicine concluded that programs aimed at decreasing the incidence of low birth weight could more effectively improve infant-mortality rates than neonatal intensive-care units. Artificial hearts are a more expensive and less effective means of improving the overall cardiovascular health of the nation than a campaign to convince people to take their high-blood-pressure medications as prescribed would be. The childproof cap for medicine bottles is a more effective approach to accidental poisonings than intensive-care units for children who have ingested the stuff. Yet we continue to give the majority of our financial support to technology-intensive care for the critically ill.

Throughout history, in fact, advances in personal medical care have generally had less impact upon overall health status than advances in public health did. Many of our greatest health advances have come from improvements in nutrition, sanitation, family planning, housing, and education. In London in 1854, Sir John Snow studied an outbreak of cholera. He noticed that everyone who came down with the disease had one thing in common: they had all obtained their drinking water from the same outdoor well. His public-health intervention was as effective as it was simple: he removed the pump handle so that no one could obtain the contaminated water. His solution was not a medical one in that it was not based on an understanding of cholera as a disease process or even of its treatment, yet it had a profound impact on health status.

It turns out that many of our most effective medical treatments were not actually introduced until *after* the diseases they cure had already begun to decline. That is, many medical advances seem to *follow* rather than *precede* a drop in the incidence of the diseases they combat.[27] Pneumonia was kill-ing fewer and fewer people in the years immediately before the introduction of the sulfonamide drugs in 1937. Tuberculosis deaths in England had declined before streptomycin and other antituberculosis agents came upon the scene in the 1940s. Going even farther back in history, the death rate from smallpox had already dropped dramatically when Jenner discovered how to immunize people against it in 1798. These medical breakthroughs further reduced deaths from these diseases to be sure, i.e., they did have an incremental effect on mortality, but they did not make as great a contribution as we tend to think.

Why were these infectious diseases already declining? Beginning in the early eighteenth century, people's nutrition began improving, with more balanced diets and less starvation. Public sanitation and personal hygiene improved from the mid-nineteenth century on (through advances such as water purification and chlorination, the pasteurization and bottling of milk, sanitary engineering and sewage disposal, and more careful handling and storage of food), thus lowering the incidence of water- and food-borne diseases. Improvements in living and working conditions, including the ventilation of closed spaces, were also important. At a time when the five leading causes of death were infectious and microbial, the introduction of these public-health measures initiated a steady decrease in mortality. The subsequent introduction of new medical treatments then produced additional decrements.

The point of all this is that personal medical care is actually somewhat less effective in improving health than we tend to think, and this discrepancy between our expectations and reality makes us ripe for disenchantment with the medical-care system.

Medical Care Causes Disease

There is another paradox in the medicalization of contemporary America: the more diseases we treat, the more disorders we create. A small but significant proportion of diagnostic procedures and medical treatments harm patients through unintended adverse consequences and negative side effects. These are called iatrogenic disorders, meaning that they are caused by the medical intervention itself. Iatrogenic disorders include such things as postoperative infections and allergic reactions to X-ray dyes. In one study, 36 percent of hospitalized patients were found to have developed at least one iatrogenic illness.[28] In one-quarter of these people (9 percent of all the hospitalized patients), these iatrogenic illnesses were of major proportions, and in 2 percent of all the patients admitted, the iatrogenic illness contributed directly to the death of the patient. Drug reactions are a common source of iatrogenic illness: serious adverse drug reactions are estimated to occur in 15 percent of hospitalized patients. Since patients now receive more medications than they used to, harmful drug side effects are increasingly common.

History reveals a number of medical innovations that were introduced with high hopes and great promise, but that ultimately resulted in great iatrogenic harm. Retrolental fibroplasia is a form of blindness that was produced in newborns who received high levels of oxygen in their incubators as a treatment for severe lung disease.[29] The drug Thalidomide, widely prescribed to treat the nausea of pregnancy, produced severe congenital defects in thousands of babies born to mothers who had taken it.

But DES (diethylstilbestrol) is the classic case in point, and an instructive one when considering the paradoxical results of the pursuit of health. After its introduction in 1938, the use of DES spread on the wings of our euphoria about the benefits of administering hormones, which we had just learned to isolate and synthesize in the laboratory.[30] DES was originally prescribed to prevent miscarriage, and for toxemia of pregnancy, a serious medical disorder, but its use was subsequently broadened from the treatment of specific disorders to the enhancement of the quality of life. It was given to suppress lactation in mothers who did not wish to nurse their babies; it was prescribed for hot flashes in post-menopausal women, and consequently seemed to be a way of slowing aging.[31] It was not until later that we discovered its terrible association with cancer in the daughters of women who took it.

DES points out both the seriousness of iatrogenic illness and the dangers of "treating" conditions that are not diseases. The indications for prescribing DES widened because of an evolution in our understanding of the goals of medicine. As R. J. Apfel and S. M. Fisher describe in their careful study of DES, "Medicine's traditional goal—to assist the natural processes of life and healing—was replaced with the notion that the forces of nature themselves are subject to control. DES became a means by which life itself could be mastered. It could help create life, then maintain youth and inhibit aging."[32]

The potential for causing harm is inherent in the process of medical care and is thus to be expected and accepted. But it must also be respected, especially when we medicalize conditions that are not serious or are not even disorders at all. As medical care becomes more ambitious and more aggressive, serious iatrogenic disorders are more likely to occur. In applying medical treatments to an ever-widening spectrum of human problems, we must be sure that these treatments are beneficial, and that the conditions being treated are serious enough to merit potential risks . . . because the price we pay can indeed be high. When we greet apparent medical advances with unbridled enthusiasm and lack of caution, when we are too eager to await more definitive evaluation of their efficacy, when we begin to believe that medicine can change the course of nature itself, we are ripe for an unsatisfactory result.

Benjamin Franklin observed, "Nothing is more fatal to health than an overcare of it." The potential for unintended harm is inherent in the very nature of all medical treatment.

We have seen in this section that increments in medical care can be unrewarding and, upon rare occasion, even harmful. Once we have achieved a high standard of personal medical care, further improvements in that care have a declining impact on overall health status. Yet there are still benefits to be derived from advances in public health and in the delivery of medical care to underserved groups.

The Paradoxical Pursuit of Wellness

Casualities of the Fitness Boom

Regular, moderate exercise is beneficial. It lowers the risk of several diseases, helps keep weight under control, and may even increase life expectancy for some.[33] But the pursuit of fitness has negative consequences as well.

Exercise-related injuries and accidents are obvious examples. Indeed, we have had to develop an entire medical specialty, sports medicine, just to repair all the damage we inflict upon ourselves in the name of fitness. (The sales of first-aid products have also skyrocketed, in large part due to an increase in sports-related injuries.)[34] Dr. James Nicholas, director of the Institute of Sports Medicine and Athletic Trauma, estimates that there are 17 to 20 million sports injuries in the U.S. each year.[35] Many take the slogan "no pain, no gain" literally, although it is false, and believe they must push themselves until their bodies ache in order to benefit from exercise.

Most hard-core runners eventually suffer injuries to their knees, ankles, backs, or feet, and one-third of women marathoners surveyed reported stress fractures.[36] A year of running has been estimated to entail a one-in-ten chance of sustaining an injury serious enough to require medical attention.[37] Nor is running the only dangerous exercise. In 1984, hospital emergency rooms treated people for 18,000 injuries related to the use of exercise equipment.[38] Aerobics too causes casualties, and although most are not serious, the

American College of Obstetrics and Gynecology has become concerned enough to urge less intensive and less frequent workouts.

For some, exercise is grim and deadly serious, a kind of physical therapy. Conditioning can become an addiction, an irresistible imperative. The problem, like that of workaholism, is not the goal pursued, but the exclusivity and single-mindedness with which it is pursued. Exercise addicts might play an hour of handball, follow it with a vigorous workout on weight-training equipment, and finish with a ten-mile run. Many acknowledge that their pursuit has taken on a compulsive quality. Unable to modify their regimen even if ill or injured, they somehow come to be dominated by the drive to exercise. One such marathoner, who never altered his regimen on account of the weather, ran along a heavily traveled road in a nasty sleet storm one February night. As passing trucks splashed him from head to toe, he became nauseated by the taste of the road salt dissolved in the slush that showered him. Yet on he trudged. A leading fitness magazine cautions the nighttime jogger to wear a cap with reflective yarn in it, running shoes with light-reflecting trim, glow-in-the-dark strips at ankles and wrists, and to carry a flashlight in each hand. If it is really that dangerous, should we be out there in the first place? And if it is not dangerous, why take it so seriously?

Compulsive runners are often men in their thirties and forties, self-effacing, hardworking, high achievers from upper-middle-class backgrounds. Running is a way of life for them, an entire personal identity complete with books, magazines, rituals, clothing, diaries, and the company of friends of similar bent.[39] The compulsive runners who have been studied seem to be uncomfortable with their emotions and inhibited in their expression of feelings, and they have often turned to running at a time in their lives when they are under great emotional stress. They are extraordinarily weight conscious and often very thin. In this respect, there are some similarities between compulsive runners and women suffering from anorexia nervosa.[40]

Strenuous exercise may literally be addictive because of a reaction it trips off in the brain. Research suggests that prolonged exercise prompts the brain to release substances called endorphins, which are potent painkillers, in effect our own, intrinsic narcotic, manufactured in the brain. This may be why long-distance runners seem to become insensitive to weakness and pain. Endorphins have another effect as well: they cause euphoria and elation, similar to the "rush" experienced by people using narcotics. The much discussed "runner's high" may be due to a sudden release of endorphins triggered by intense exercise, resulting in a chemically induced state so pleasurable that it is addicting.

There is an additional negative consequence of the exercise boom. Physical conditioning can become an excuse for withdrawing from the real world into oneself. Little time or interest remains for work, family, or even for sex. Rather than remaining one element of a complete life, exercise becomes a substitute for everything else. The tail comes to wag the dog. Some fitness fanatics change jobs in order to have enough time to exercise, or break up with lovers who don't work out as much. As Dr. George Sheehan, author and apostle of running, has said, "Jobs, family, friends will wait . . . can anything have a higher priority than running?"[41] Sheehan, for example, ultimately came to see himself as a runner, rather than as a doctor, husband, father, or friend. Like hypochondriacs, these compulsive athletes are more interested in their bodies and their performance than in anything else.

These are the casualties of the fitness boom: people who suffer orthopedic damage or develop a kind of personal addiction that leads them to withdraw from the real world. This happens when physical conditioning acquires deeper psychological meanings and stands for something far more than mere muscle tone and cardiovascular health.

Casualties of the Dieting Boom

The situation with respect to the dieting boom is similar. Much of the current emphasis upon diet is beneficial, in that nutrition and weight control are important in health and their roles have been underappreciated until recently. But here, too, there are some negative consequences that we would do well to bear in mind.

For one thing, stringent fad diets are harmful. The World Health Organization defines starvation as a daily intake of less than 1,000 calories, so many of these dieters are literally starving themselves. Are these Spartan diets nutritionally unsound? Yes. For one thing, they are deficient in essential nutrients. And sadly, this has even become a problem for infants and toddlers. Pediatricians have begun seeing children whose growth has been retarded because they were placed on stringent low-fat, low-calorie diets by well-meaning parents overly concerned about dietary cholesterol and childhood obesity.[42] In addition to their nutritional deficiencies, fad diets are dangerous in other ways. Some, for example, can cause sudden and even fatal disturbances in heart rhythm. Or they lead to a pattern of rapid weight loss and regain, which is more deleterious to health than remaining consistently overweight. (The very notion of a crash diet is intrinsically fallacious because time-limited, draconian efforts to lose many pounds in a brief period do not succeed in the long run.)

There is another harmful facet of the weight-loss craze. It is contagious, and some people who catch it are unable to keep the powerful social pressures to be thin in perspective. Two such vulnerable groups are young children and people predisposed to eating disorders. Our obsession with dieting has infected the sixty-pound weight class: 80 percent of fourth-grade girls in San Francisco believe they weigh too much and are dieting, according to a University of California study.[43] The same yearning to be thin was found in a survey of fourth-grade girls in Chicago, more than half of whom had dieted. Many were terrified of gaining weight and kept their dieting secret from their parents.[44] By dieting, these children risk stunting their growth as well as developing nutritional deficiencies and eating disorders.

Some people become so obsessed with being thin that they develop an uncontrollable compulsion to diet. We are witnessing a dramatic rise in the prevalence of a psychiatric eating disorder called anorexia nervosa. Anorexic women (for the disease afflicts mostly women) are horrified by obesity and have a distorted perception of their bodies as being fat, even though in fact they are emaciated. Anorexics diet so stringently that they literally starve themselves, even to death in 10 percent of cases. An anorexic, for example, might eat two or three peas for dinner, cutting each up into quarters with a knife and fork before slowly chewing and swallowing the pieces individually.

The anorexic's horror of obesity and pursuit of thinness seem to be an extreme version of the general dieting craze. We do not know what causes anorexia, but the increasing incidence of this disorder in the last fifteen years is thought to be related to the increasing social pressure to be thin during this period. This theory is supported by the finding that anorexia is more common among women who are under exceptional pressure to be thin, such as fashion models and ballet dancers, than it is among other women of comparable age and social class.[45] And many models and dancers who are not frankly anorexic exhibit some of the features of the disorder, such as a distorted body image, excessive dieting, and vomiting to control weight.[46] Some observers have suggested that the more stringent popular diets function as a kind of training ground for eating disorders. For example, the Beverly Hills Diet actually prescribes a disordered pattern of binging and starving like that seen in the eating disorder bulimia.[47]

Casualties of the Mass Media's Focus on Health

As we have noted, the mass communications media feature health and medicine prominently. Many of their educational and instructional efforts produce a more knowledgeable and better educated citizenry who become more enlightened medical consumers. Many people are thereby enabled to take better care of themselves—but there are also some negative side effects.

The media's efforts sometimes foster a sense of insecurity about health, which amplifies feelings of ill health. In the race for attention, promotion, and a wider audience, the media employ a kind of medical hyperbole. The risks of potential health hazards are sometimes exaggerated; serious factual inaccuracies may be relayed to the public; tentative research findings are blown out of proportion and portrayed as fact, touted as major breakthroughs before any confirmatory evidence is in hand.[48] This "medico-media hype,"[49] promulgated by the media, advertising, public relations, manufacturers, and some members of the health professions, makes health a source of apprehension in the minds of some. These people are excessively frightened by reports (many exaggerated) of new and dreadful diseases. Because of the publicity devoted to Alzheimer's disease, for instance, it has recently become necessary to reassure the public that forgetfulness is common and usually normal.[50] Misinformation and the resulting confusion lead people to seek medical care needlessly and make them vulnerable to quacks who "treat" them at great expense for disorders that they do not have or that do not even exist. Medico-media hype also sometimes raises false hopes and expectations in people with incurable diseases, holding out the prospect of new miracle cures that do not exist.

No matter how well-meaning the media's attempts to inform and protect the public are, the result is sometimes a lamentable increase in confusion and misinformation. A great deal of media attention has been focused upon the alarming rise in suicide among the young, for example. But studies show that this coverage actually aggravates the problem: teenagers commit suicide in greater numbers following television news programs or feature stories about adolescent suicide. And surprisingly, this happens after sober and constructive programs that address the problem in general, as much as it does following sensationalized and shocking stories about the suicides of particular people.[51]

The scare over toxic-shock syndrome exemplifies the way in which public warnings about a medical problem can generate disproportionate public anxiety.[52] Toxic-shock syndrome, a rare infection, was thrust into the public awareness in 1980 and 1981 after an obscure medical report was widely publicized in the mass media. When a single study raised the possibility that the syndrome might be linked to a specific brand of tampon (it is not, in fact), toxic-shock syndrome became a household word and the Rely tampon became the culprit. There was national coverage in the nightly news, and in only four months, millions were terrified, products were recalled, and lawsuits were filed.[53]

The media covered the story intensively: a mysterious, fatal disease was striking healthy young women and might be due to a widely used product. Criticized for turning the disease into "toxic-schlock syndrome," the coverage was handled as part detective story, part disaster story, concentrating on the human-interest angle at the expense of the scientific facts.[54] This hyperbole overplayed the magnitude of the danger. While it is an important public-health threat and a serious, even fatal, disease, toxic-shock syndrome is nevertheless relatively rare and not nearly as lethal as was popularly concluded.* For the many healthy women who felt feverish and worried, the mass media's coverage of this issue resulted in feelings of ill health.

---

* Most victims do not die of the disease but instead recover fully. Actual rates are unclear, but there are probably about 5,000 cases per year, or 9 out of 100,000 menstruating women.[55]

As the anorexic is a casualty of our horror of obesity, and the compulsive runner a casualty of our obsession with fitness, so people with "total allergy syndrome" and "ecological illness" may be casualties of media stories about "environmental allergies." These allergies supposedly result from synthetic chemicals in the environment. In response to wide media coverage, more and more people began complaining that they were "environmentally ill," globally allergic to common, everyday substances.[56] In severe cases, these patients feel incapable of living in the modern world, believing they have life-threatening allergies to soap, carpets, clothing, furniture, even water. One such patient notes, "For example, churches, unfortunately, tend to provide a particularly poor ecological environment. They tend to be closed during the week, holding in fumes and generating musty atmospheres; they tend to be tenderly cared for with new carpets and paints and frequent cleanings which release chlorine and alcohols into the air; they tend to draw people, particularly on Sunday morning, who wear their newest clothes and their finest perfumes which introduce formalin and phenol into an already well-contaminated ecology." Careful medical investigation has failed to demonstrate any such disease as global "environmental allergies." While people may be allergic to specific substances, such as dust or pollen or animal hair, they do not usually suffer from anything so generalized. Rather, it seems that these people have been coaxed into feelings of dis-ease, or into expressing their dis-ease in this way, by the publicity and hoopla spawned by the media.

The Psychological Paradox

The pursuit of healthiness can be psychologically counterproductive as well, because heightened health consciousness can lead to a more negative assessment of health. We've discussed this point at several places in the book, but it is useful to gather the information all together here, in the context of our discussion of various sorts of paradoxes. A broad psychological principle that is relevant here is that the more aware a person becomes of his characteristics and attributes, the more negatively he will assess them. This is especially true of one's physical characteristics and perceptions of health; chances are, the more you study the shape of your nose in the mirror, the less you will like it. Thus America's intense interest in health may in and of itself lead many individuals to become less satisfied with their own health.

We also know that the more introspective and self-conscious you become, the more you will be troubled by mild and inconsequential bodily sensations. Paying more attention to your body causes you to notice sensations that you ignored or dismissed in the past. And the more bodily symptoms you perceive, the more alarmed you become about your health. This alarm then prompts further self-scrutiny, during which you will surely note additional sensations that you had not noticed before. Now, in the context of a rising concern about your health, these symptoms seem more ominous and more intense, making you more likely to conclude that they are due to a serious disease rather than to something harmless. A vicious cycle is created in which self-consciousness begets symptoms, symptoms produce alarm, and alarm heightens self-consciousness even further.

As a society, we seem to be caught in this vicious cycle. Our heightened health consciousness and our national mood of dis-ease furnish an ominous backdrop against which we view our health and try to decipher our somatic sensations. The constant warnings that every bodily experience might be the first sign of cancer or angina or AIDS direct our attention ever more insistently to our bodies and give us additional reasons to pore over our symptoms. This brings about a more negative appraisal of our health. We notice trivial illnesses and amplify troublesome ones. The medicalization of everyday life and the belief in personal control of health have the same result. The culturally induced pursuit of health backfires, leaving us ill at ease and symptomatic.

We discussed an additional psychological paradox earlier: equating health with "healthy" behavior and practices makes some people feel unhealthy merely because they are not following these prescribed and proscribed activities, even when they are actually perfectly healthy.[57] The failure to take active steps to preserve our health leaves us feeling ill at ease because we are violating certain taboos for which, we are warned, we will pay a price subsequently.

Our fear of stress can produce a similar result. It is not just that we must avoid stressful events, but that we must control our personal reactions to them. Wellness requires that we maintain a positive mental outlook and a relaxed attitude toward life's crises and pressures. We must be able to banish disturbing thoughts from our minds. "Take things easy!," "Relax!," "Stop worrying!" . . . or else you will make yourself sick. But then the injunction, the command not to worry, itself becomes arduous.[58] Just keeping up with all the medical news about what is harmful raises our stress levels, filling us with an even greater sense of effort and struggle. The paradoxical effect is that striving and straining to relax only upsets us further, bringing about the very state we are laboring so hard to conquer.

Curable Pain Is Unbearable Pain: The Problem of Rising Expectations

Pain that we believe can be *assuaged,* that we think is *unnecessary,* hurts more than pain that is *unavoidable* and *inevitable.*[59] The only thing as bad as pain itself is waiting for it to end, for relief we believe is imminent. Say you lie waiting for the codeine you've just taken to numb the pain of a scratched cornea; once you expect the pain to go away, as soon as you think enough time has passed for you to be feeling better, the pain seems even more excruciating, and you don't think you can endure one more minute.

With chronic symptoms, something similar happens: when you believe that an infirmity is treatable, it seems more burdensome and more severe. Once you believe that your arthritic hands should not hurt as much as they do, that relief would be forthcoming if only you could find the right specialist or get hold of the latest experimental drug, then the aching and the stiffness become intolerable. Thinking that a cure for your condition exists but has eluded you prevents you from learning to cope with your distress and minimize it. It is only when we accept the fact that some of our ailments are inescapable, that some afflictions are unavoidable, that we can learn how to put up with them and get on with the business of living.

Thus, studies of facial deformities and disfigurements show that minor deviations cause as much or more mental anguish than defects too major to be corrected.[60] It is agonizing to feel that you are almost, but not quite, normal. Some people like this become obsessed with their appearance, going to inordinate expense and effort to eliminate the problem. On the other hand, more grossly deformed or handicapped individuals have had to accept their defects and thus have learned how to cope with them.[61]

Studies of obesity suggest something similar. Overweight people who are trying to reduce are more unhappy than overweight people who have accepted their condition and are not trying to lose weight.[62] Dieting and becoming weight conscious in themselves seem to make some people more unhappy about their weight. Perhaps feeling that a normal weight is within the realm of possibility but failing to attain it is more disturbing than never having aspired to thinness in the first place; once you admit how much you dislike your size and you have tried hard to alter it, it becomes intolerable. An alternative explanation for these findings is that the people who try to reduce are more unhappy to begin with, and the people who are more content never try to diet. The finding, however, is not explained by supposing that those trying to lose weight are fatter to start with and are more unhappy for that reason, since all of the people studied are of comparable weight—about 20 percent above average.

Our society's quest for health produces the kind of frustration expressed in these examples because of our belief that we control our own health, and because of the growing medicalization of our society. These forces convey the idea that more and more kinds of suffering and misery are curable. They lead us to expect that almost every pain is treatable, every infirmity is avoidable, and that every remedy is guaranteed to work. One need look no further than our advertising: "Rolaids spells relief," "Murine adds nothing but relief," and so on. Nearsightedness, weariness, dry skin, as well as cancer and senility and heart attacks, are all supposed to melt away with the proper medication or procedure.

Everyday life is supposed to be symptom-free, devoid of discomfort or malaise, "Because you never get tired of feeling good."[63] The prospect of a pain-free, ailment-free life appears to be at hand. "Get rid of pain forever," proclaims Bonnie Prudden in her latest book. She promises "a safe, drug-free way to eliminate pain caused by stress, accidents, sports, disease, and job hazards. [With] Bonnie Prudden's total program for lifelong fitness, health, and freedom from pain . . . you can enjoy pain-free living *and* slow down the aging process."[64] We have always *aspired* to control our health; what is new about our era is the *belief* that we can do it, that we are on the threshold of eliminating sickness and suffering as categories of human experience.

And so the foundation is laid for dissatisfaction and disappointment with our health. People are so inculcated with the notion that a successful treatment exists for whatever ails them that they experience the persistence of symptoms as a failure of their medical care, some kind of mistake. Unrealistic optimism makes it harder for us to live with the mishaps and miseries that are not in fact curable. We expect such great success in our pursuit of wellness that we are bound to be disillusioned by our actual health, as good as it is. The ultimate discovery that we cannot really control our medical fate comes as a rude shock since we had thought we could, and it makes medicine's shortcomings seem insufferable.

An analogy with the automobile suggests itself. Think of the impatience and discontent that the automobile's great promise of speed and freedom generate while we sit in a traffic jam. Getting stuck behind the wheel in a congested area is distressing because it runs counter to our heightened expectations.[65] It is a paradox: the potential for great speed increases our displeasure with having to go slowly. This same displeasure seems to be engendered by the pace of medical research. Every news report containing the slightest hint of an advance in the therapy of some serious disease unleashes a flood of requests for it from frantic sufferers,[66] but since the treatment is still only experimental, it is unavailable on a mass scale. Patients become angry and desperate, feeling that lifesaving therapies are being unjustifiably denied them, suspecting that other people with more money or more clout are somehow getting the coveted treatment.

If we undertake it with unrealistic expectations, then our quest for wellness may result not in greater feelings of healthiness, but in greater dis-ease. Raising our hopes too high can backfire, making our ultimate illnesses and infirmities more difficult to bear than they otherwise would have been.

In Summary

Our society's fervent pursuit of health has made us the healthiest society ever. But it has not been accompanied by a feeling of physical well-being and vigor. The problem is that the healthier we become, the more concerned with health we become. Indeed, people now seem to be more troubled by benign symptoms and more disabled by mild illnesses than they used to be.

Medicalization stimulates the fantasy that suffering and disease can eventually be eliminated, but this is illusory: they are threads woven throughout the tapestry of human existence. Disease is inextricably intertwined with health; aging is not a disease that can be treated; death is not an event that can be postponed indefinitely. Indeed, the nature of medical interventions is such that they actually increase the proportion of people who are chronically impaired. Even physical fitness, sound nutrition, health education, and expertise in self-care can have negative consequences when a sense of moderation and proportion is lost and these things are taken to extremes.

The quest for health can also become counterproductive because thinking, talking, and reading about health so much can undermine feelings of well-being. The war on disease can result in dis-ease by raising anxiety and alarm and by making us more sensitive to our inevitable aches and pains. It is impossible to feel healthy when every discomfort merits medical attention, when every twinge seems to herald a serious disease, when every wrinkle and sag and mole deserves surgery.

Because our dream is so alluring and our ambitions are set so high, our efforts almost inevitably leave us feeling disenchanted. Our dedication to the proposition that all disease is treatable and all suffering remediable makes untreatable pain and incurable illness intolerable. An unhealed ulcer or a chronic backache is worse when unrealistic fantasies of cure have been dashed and our expectations disappointed; now we feel cheated and frustrated, as well as ill.

CHAPTER 10

You Can't Feel Healthy Without Feeling Sick

IT IS POSSIBLE to reap the benefits of medical progress without feeling dis-eased at the same time. But this requires facing the reality of illness and accepting it, since it is not possible to feel truly healthy and hardy without also knowing what it is to be sick.

Calcium Supplements Won't Make Life More Fulfilling

Physical health is not the same thing as happiness, optimism, satisfaction with life, or self-fulfillment. We need to be clear about just what we can, and cannot, expect to result from the pursuit of health. Taking calcium supplements, having a normal electrocardiogram, even living longer, do not necessarily mean that we will experience a greater sense of self-worth. Walking up stairs instead of taking the elevator and substituting bran flakes for eggs are good things to do, as long as we don't expect them to help us love what we are doing more or become better at it. It is an illusion that controlling our health means controlling our lives. Successful living can't be reduced to a health problem, and good health will never satisfy our longings for other important things we need. On the contrary, unrealistic expectations of wellness leave us ripe for dismay and resentment when we find that all our efforts and sacrifices have not brought the personal and emotional returns we dreamed of.

Likewise, it is important not to let our fears get the best of us. People have a terrible propensity for bringing about the very thing they fear most in all the world. The husband who is terrified that his wife will one day stop loving him hovers over her and smothers her with attention, stifling her because of his insecurity; finally, she feels so imprisoned that she leaves him and files for divorce. The mother frightened that her daughter will be anything less than an academic superstar pressures the child unmercifully, making her feel inadequate; her daughter's anxiety makes her do poorly and she ultimately drops out of school. People may try to avoid something so intently that in the end they bring it about. If you are terribly afraid of getting sick, you may spend so much time stamping out every hint of discomfort, and being dominated by the health implications of everything you do, that you end up living the life of an invalid.

Understanding Personal Health Concerns as Metaphors

The Personal Meanings of Health and Illness

Physical well-being is overvalued whenever it symbolizes other human needs. Confusing good health with a more fulfilling and satisfying life is a sure sign that deeper personal concerns are masquerading as health concerns. Early in the book we saw that people use bodily metaphors to articulate psychological distress, that they become preoccupied with their physical health when they are actually worried about themselves as people. We also saw that the same thing can happen to a culture: practices, beliefs, and attitudes about health can be metaphors for deeper cultural problems, such as powerlessness, disintegration, and narcissism.

George Chase's reaction to illness illustrates the way in which health concerns camouflage deeper personal concerns. George, a management consultant, and his wife, Caroline, were both enthralled with "life in the fast lane." George had always been very assertive and wanted to "win" at everything he did. He found it almost impossible to relax, since he would immediately begin thinking about "more productive things" he should be doing with his time. He worked long hours and traveled frequently on business. His motto was "If you're not last onto the airplane, you've been wasting time." When not working, he was either jogging or remodeling their large house.

At the age of thirty-seven, George developed diabetes. Initially, he couldn't believe it was true, so he didn't take his insulin carefully. Then, when it finally sank in, he became hypochondriacal. He developed headaches, and hearing about the dangers of lead poisoning on television, he decided that this was the source of his symptoms, since he had stripped old paint from the walls while remodeling his house. He felt so sick in general that it was "impossible to give 110 percent," and his work suffered. Caroline found him increasingly irritable and despondent, and she convinced him to see a psychiatrist, though he was ashamed and very reluctant to go.

George felt driven to succeed in his job, and he viewed his health and his body as valuable assets in his climb to the top. As he said, "I may not be smarter than most of my competitors, but I can beat them by working harder and being better prepared." Until he got diabetes, George had always imagined that his capacity for hard work was unlimited, that his body would perform no matter how many meals he skipped, or how little sleep he got, or how much pressure he was under. His illness therefore devastated him, because he could no longer take his health and his body for granted; for the first time he encountered real physical limitations on how much he could do. His illness signified to him the loss of his most important assets: his stamina, his fortitude, his drive.

In psychotherapy, George came to understand himself better and learned what having diabetes meant to him. He began to acknowledge the inevitability of constraints even in a healthy life, understanding that there were indeed limits to how much work he could do or how many hours he could squeeze out of a single day or how fast he could run. Accepting this reality allowed him to take some measure of pride in his accomplishments, rather than judging them against an unrealistically high ideal. Always a serious runner, he began comparing his times with those of others his age rather than against world records. As he learned to accept his personal limitations, he learned to accept his physical limitations and then his illness. He noted, "When I'm feeling stronger about myself, it's a little easier to face that I have a health problem."

We each prize good health, but for different reasons. The meaning of illness—what is most frightening about it, what it deprives us of, what aspect of it is most dreadful—is astonishingly unpredictable and variable from one person to another. A graduate student in history, who had gone blind from glaucoma three years earlier, answered an inquiry about what her illness had been like with the startling admission, "Going blind was the best thing that ever happened to me." Blindness legitimized her dependence on friends and relatives, something she had always felt but that had seemed unacceptable and shameful before she became disabled.

Everyone is disturbed by sickness, of course, but some are disturbed because they fear it will result in abandonment by others, some because it means they will not live long enough to reach a personal milestone, some because it makes them feel as if they are being punished for something they did. Sickness makes some people feel like failures, while it makes others feel weak and helpless, or unloved, or out of control.

This sort of self-knowledge helps lessen the paradoxical dis-ease that can come with the pursuit of wellness. Knowing the private meanings we attach to good health protects us against disappointment, unfulfilled expectations, and dashed hopes even as we remain healthy; it saves us from the dismay of discovering that our wish to feel more confident about the future isn't fulfilled by stockpiling our own blood for a rainy day, that a feeling of personal inadequacy isn't quashed by learning to do cardiopulmonary resuscitation.

In addition, such self-knowledge gives us more control over our lives because we now have a better picture of what things are most important to us and what things are most frightening. Knowing this, we can try to deal with our concerns directly, rather than in disguised form such as concerns about cancer or calcium or cholesterol. If good health is important to you because it means being more attractive and desirable to others, you would do better to focus upon your own sense of attractiveness and desirability. For such people feeling lovable is the issue that deserves their attention, not their physical health. If you fear illness most because you can't stand the idea of depending upon other people, of being at someone else's mercy, you would be better served by learning to trust and rely on others than by checking your blood pressure again or rereading the *Merck Manual.* If you prize good health most because it makes you feel blessed, more favored, and more special than others, you need to learn to feel better about yourself as a person, not as a physical specimen. Thus, self-knowledge permits us to pursue our real goals directly and to work on the problems that are really disturbing us, rather than ineffectually focusing on the health concerns and preoccupations that mask what's really on our minds.

Sickness and Solitude

Loneliness is one of the most powerful and most universal personal meanings of illness. "As sickness is the greatest misery," said John Donne, "so the greatest misery of sickness is solitude." Illness is a state of solitary confinement: with every illness, infectious or not, comes a quarantine of sorts. Lying awake at night awaiting the results of a biopsy for cancer, or finding one can no longer read because of deteriorating vision—these are intensely private experiences. So the sick, in addition to their physical suffering, endure the psychological suffering of loneliness. Illness secludes us by making us different from others; it underscores our ultimate separateness. No matter how empathic the people around us are, no matter how loving or how solicitous, it is the afflicted individual alone who endures the frustration of being rendered mute by a stroke, the pain of a kidney stone, the mutilation of a mastectomy.

Mankind's two greatest miseries are the physical pain of injury or sickness and the mental pain of separation from our loved ones, especially their loss. The intimate relationship between physical suffering and loneliness has always been recognized. Throughout the Bible, for example, a connection is repeatedly made between being "cut off " from others and being diseased.[1] This is exemplified by Job, upon whom God visits the worst possible trials: the physical suffering of sickness and the psychological suffering of losing his children.[2] Physical affliction and interpersonal isolation are woven together into a single tapestry of anguish.

People tend to pull back, to withdraw, from the sick because it is so sad and so frightening to be with them. In addition, the sick person himself becomes selfish and self-centered. He is preoccupied with his discomfort and withdraws into himself, retreating from the outside world back into the wounded confines of his body. Formerly important characters are now demoted to the status of bit players, drifting through the background of a drama in which the sick person alone occupies center stage. Think back to Frank Carson's day. Everyone he dealt with, from his wife to his co-workers, was subsidiary. Each was eclipsed by the shadow of disease that had fallen across Frank's world. His fears and his symptoms were dominant, making everything else pale.

There is another, and contrary, aspect of the relationship between sickness and solitude. For although illness secludes you, at the very same time it also draws people to you. Sickness galvanizes those around you into helping you, mobilizing them and bringing them to your side. As we've seen, one of the most basic of all human equations, learned in earliest infancy, is that pain brings love. It follows then that to tell someone about your pain is to ask for their help.[3] Thus we found that hypochondriacs are often expressing feelings of loneliness and isolation through their feelings of illness. A false alarm about health can be set off in all of us when important relationships are jeopardized.

Understanding Societal Health Concerns as Metaphors

America's obsession with health and disease both expresses and disguises several themes that are less tangible but no less important. In searching for these deeper cultural themes behind our society's health concerns, the preceding discussion would point us first toward sources of interpersonal estrangement and social isolation; it would suggest that we search for rents in the social fabric that are in need of repair.

Social Estrangement

The social institutions that in the past helped people to bear suffering and cope with sickness are in decline. Declines in the neighborhood, the extended family, and the religious community, and our estrangement from each other, are a source of cultural hypochondria. We need social support and social integration—we need other human beings—in order to withstand sickness, old age, and death. As interpersonal estrangement grows, as people have become more isolated from each other, we have grown increasingly fearful of illness, that most isolating of all human experiences. Our preoccupation with health signals a weakening of the web of social support that is spun by the family, the community, and even by the casual assistance of strangers. We worry about falling ill, and it is more awful when we become ill because we don't feel as if people care about us or care for us, because we feel too estranged from neighbors, extended family, coworkers.

But, just as we saw with individuals, our society's increased health consciousness expresses more than people's distance from each other; it is, at the same time, an attempt to remedy the problem, to nurture greater cohesion. Societal hypochondria is in part a call for help, a way of countering the self-centeredness and narcissism and interpersonal isolation that are afoot. In proclaiming a state of emergency, we hope to get others' attention, to startle others out of their indifference to us. The fitness movement exemplifies this, since it is a means of social identification and affiliation, and since working out is a ritual that can be shared and performed with others. Health clubs have replaced the sewing circle and the dance; they are places to make friends. The self-help movement is likewise a group movement, one based on mutual aid and support, shared experiences, and the establishment of close relationships among group members. Thus, self-help groups like Reach for Recovery, Parents without Partners, and Al-Anon replace the small-town social network, the close-knit neighborhood of bygone times.

The Fear of Interdependency

Independence, individualism, and autonomy are among America's most cherished ideals.[4] Think of the self-reliant cowboy in the western movie, alone but totally self-sufficient, beholden to no one, dependent upon no one. Independence also lies at the heart of the free-enterprise system. It is exemplified by do-it-yourself home projects, the self-service store, and mail-order kits to prepare your own divorce or will. Our affluence and technology have been employed to minimize our interdependence: we watch a movie on a VCR at home rather than sitting with others in a movie theater; we drive to work in our own cars rather than joining with strangers on a bus or a train; we buy a private house in the suburbs rather than renting an apartment in the city. Even within the family we seek to maximize separateness and individuality: each member strives for his own television, his own room, his own telephone, even his own car. We have private airplanes, private boxes at sports stadiums, private lessons for our children. To be sure, only the very wealthy can have these privacies, but they reveal what we aspire to.

In the realm of health as well, we strive to maximize autonomy, independence, and self-sufficiency. As we saw in chapter 7, the concept of wellness is inextricably bound up with the doctrines of self-control and self-reliance. For some people the fitness movement offers not a ready-made social matrix, but rather a means of honing their bodies into such durable and reliable machines that they will never need anyone to repair them; it is like learning to do your own automotive maintenance work so that you will never need a mechanic. Total fitness, it is imagined, will liberate us from having to depend on anyone else for survival. The new self-diagnostic kits, the imperative to educate oneself about the body, and the self-care movement aim to make us into autonomous medical experts who will never require a doctor's skill or assistance. This trend toward patient autonomy is also apparent in the decline of the physician's authority and our increasing mistrust of him. Indeed, the scent of a lawsuit hangs as heavy in the air of the examining room as the scent of surgical soap. Dependence upon doctors is distasteful and dangerous, so when people do become sick and have to defer to a doctor, they enter the hospital accompanied by patient advocates who stand at the ready, asserting their protection under the Patient's Bill of Rights.

But the problem is that the more autonomy and independence we achieve, the more lonely and isolated it makes us. Indeed, this sense of estrangement is part of the societal disease about health we discussed earlier in the book. Freed from the shackles of dependence upon others, we are left feeling unprotected and unsafe. It is as if we were skating alone over a deep pond covered by thin ice, unable to see anyone around to aid us should we get into trouble.

In the end we can't deny our interdependence as biological organisms and as human beings. We live out the biological programs written in our ancestors' genes; we are affected by our neighbors' cigarette smoke and our coworker's germs; we may even require someone else's kidneys to survive. Our lives, in the end, may hang upon the ministrations of a loving family, a physician's skill, or the prudence of the drivers on the highway beside us. We do depend on others for comfort when we are afraid about what will happen to us, for the care they give us when we go to bed with the flu, for their humor and mercy and generosity should we be disabled. It is even possible to die from loneliness. We ignore this human interdependency only at the risk of feeling imperiled. Because deep inside we know that we need each other when we are ill, suffering, and old. If we don't take care of each other and protect each other and watch out for each other, it ultimately erodes our feelings of physical security and well-being, heightening fears about ill health and about our ability to survive.

Our quest for wellness, then, stems in part from a rising sense of societal disintegration and from a growing fear of having to depend upon others. We fear illness so much, and we try so hard to be healthy, because we are so insecure about the interpersonal dimensions of ill health.

"To Live in Fear of Death Is to Fear Living"

Another source of our health consciousness is a declining involvement in things outside ourselves, a declining commitment to some greater good, to a cause or institution or tradition that is larger than the self. We are not a people dedicated to achieving interpersonal intimacy, or to transcending narrow self-interest, or to improving the lot of others. The question nowadays is less "What can I do?" and more "What can I get?" We are concerned most with the personal and the immediate, with what we can consume now, with how we feel and what we are experiencing at the moment. We are less interested in sublimating personal gratification and advancement for the sake of religious beliefs, a value system, a moral or spiritual code, or a historical tradition.

The more important self-interest becomes, the more important personal well-being and physical comfort become. So we now conceptualize personhood in corporeal terms, like age, appearance, fitness, stamina, and size, rather than in terms of integrity, generosity, or courage. How well the body works, how good it feels, how it looks, how long it will hold up all become paramount concerns. If there is no hereafter, no greater good, no raison d'être, then there is no rationale for tolerating discomfort or enduring disability. There is nothing more important than health, and so we must do everything possible to strengthen and preserve and protect it. Thus we are dismayed by every sign of aging, obsessed with avoiding injury and illness, disconcerted by every ache and pain.

This perspective makes death seem especially awful, and as a society we do indeed seem to be having a hard time accepting the fact of death. The problem here is that, as McCormick and Skrabanek have written in the medical journal *Lancet,* "to live in fear of death is to fear living."[5] All death, no matter what the circumstances, seems to us premature and potentially preventable. Death feels to us like an affront, an obscene mystery, a consummate evil on which we have declared war.[6] Members of the Cryonics Society (whose motto is "Never Say Die" and whose emblem is the phoenix) go so far in striving for immortality as to have themselves frozen at the point of death, to be thawed out in the future when we have a cure for whatever killed them.

We don't have the consolation of viewing death as an inevitable and inextricable part of life, as an unavoidable or even acceptable fate, the "natural" conclusion of the life cycle. We never consider that death might be welcomed by the old and infirm as sleep is welcomed by the weary. Instead, death, no matter what the timing or the circumstances, indicates a failure of some kind on someone's part. *Medical care should prevent death,* we seem to be saying. Lewis Thomas, in *The Medusa and the Snail,* speaks to this point. There is, he says, "a profound dissatisfaction with the fact of death. Dying is regarded as the ultimate failure, something that could always be avoided or averted if only the health-care system functioned more efficiently. Death has been made to seem unnatural, an outrage; when people die—at whatever age—we speak of them as having been 'struck down,' 'felled.' It is as though in a better world we would all go on forever."[7]

Many factors contribute to this extreme unease about death. One is the omnipresence and immediacy of mass nuclear destruction, what must surely be the ultimate "health hazard." As the nuclear shadow lengthens, as survival seems more and more tenuous, our fear of death is heightened. As we've seen, other aspects of contemporary life seem particularly menacing and unsafe, encircled as we are by lethal threats ranging from microwaves in our kitchens to toxic chemicals in our drinking water to commercial airplane crashes.

A blurring of the difference between being alive and being dead also fosters our unease with death. At times now, technology rather than nature regulates death; medicine can prolong dying almost indefinitely and medical care thus becomes death-delaying rather than lifesaving. Many have witnessed firsthand the modern deathbed ritual, referred to by Ivan Illich as the "sumptuous treatment of the comatose"[8]: elaborate and expensive, as protracted as it is futile, it keeps the patient alive in the technical sense even when there is no hope of meaningful recovery. An elderly widow who is senile, blind, and suffering from advanced heart and liver disease is subjected to every possible medical intervention during her final, five-week-long hospitalization. Scrubbed and neat between the clean sheets, warm and with a healthy skin color, she hardly resembles someone who is dying.[9] Prostrate in a clearing amidst a thicket of plastic tubing, she lies surrounded by winking oscilloscope screens, with wires running in and out of her body. Subspecialists glide in to consult on each organ as it gives up the ghost in turn. We seem unable to desist from intervening.[10] Each succeeding complication is met with invasive diagnostic procedures and heroic lifesaving measures. We can no longer recognize when a person's time has come.

This ability to preserve life in a vegetative state indefinitely, the capacity to sustain a dead brain in a living body, has created a new class of half-dead/half-alive people. They are not aware, and they can neither think nor feel. They lie in irreversible coma, while heart action, digestion, and metabolism are carried out indefinitely by machine. It is estimated that there are 10,000 Americans now living in such a permanent vegetative state.[11]

Similarly, when someone is going to serve as an organ donor, we continue to treat him in many respects as if he were alive, even after he has been declared dead.[12] We do not turn off the machines and send the body to the morgue. Instead we continue to monitor the patient and support his bodily functions in order to preserve the organs until they can be transplanted. This perplexing state of affairs can be terrible for the families of the patients. An article in the *New England Journal of Medicine* describes such a situation: "A little boy sitting outside the pediatric intensive care unit looked up as an older child was wheeled out on a cart, surrounded by a group of nurses and physicians. The chest of the prospective donor was moving up and down with respirations produced by a ventilator. 'That's my brother,' said the little boy. 'He's dead and they're taking him to surgery.' "[13]

The act of dying has become more disturbing because we think that medicine should be able to treat it. Instead, what we've done is to confuse the act of dying, to render it more troubling because it can be tampered with but not fixed. We have thereby raised profoundly disturbing questions about when life should end and must end.

Dealing Directly with Our Underlying Concerns

As a society, we might lessen some of our dis-ease about health if we dealt directly with the underlying concerns that are fueling it—once we see them for what they are—if we worked to build more significant interpersonal relationships and a greater sense of social integration and cohesion.

Strengthening the Cohesion of Our Society

We need to begin to redress our unhealthy level of concern for personal rather than societal well-being. If our institutions brought us *psychologically* closer together, we might be less terrified of the lonely *biological* fate awaiting us. Community projects, religious affiliation, philanthropic efforts, neighborhood activities, extended families—all help us to live with our afflictions and to bear the knowledge that we will eventually die. The hypochondriac's symptoms often abate when he establishes a meaningful personal relationship with a doctor. When he feels cared for, he worries less about falling ill. If we each felt a greater sense of community, of social support and mutual caretaking, if there were greater opportunities to live in trust, cooperation, and friendship with those around us, then our feelings of dis-ease might abate. We must nurture our resources for bearing sickness and pain, the social institutions and activities that bring us together in meaningful and cooperative ways and support us when life's difficulties visit. Neighborhood associations, retirement communities, co-ops, child-care centers, and other groups that organize for a common purpose—all help in this regard.

Strengthening our social supports certainly won't harm our health status either. Several years ago, researchers who

were raising rabbits on a special disease-producing diet noticed something puzzling. A few of the animals remained
perfectly healthy and never got sick on the diet. The only
thing different about these rabbits was that they were all
kept in cages that were about six feet off the ground—at the
researchers' eye level. It turned out that because of this, the
experimenters had been patting them and playing with them
when they fed them, and these animals were therefore getting much more attention than those whose cages were
above or below. In 1980 this was studied rigorously. Laboratory rabbits were fed a diet designed to give them athero-
sclerotic heart disease. Some of them had a one-to-one relationship with an experimenter who handled, stroked, and
played with them, while the rest did not. The first group
developed 60 percent less atherosclerosis than the rabbits
receiving usual laboratory care and the same diet.[14] When
we move from the laboratory into the real world, from animals to people, we find something similar. Isolated individuals with few close personal contacts have more physical and
mental disorders, and die earlier, than those with a network
of friends to whom they regularly turn. Married people have
lower morbidity and mortality rates than those who are wid-
owed, divorced, or single. Having a supportive spouse protects people who are undergoing stressful events. Men with
emotionally supportive wives, for example, endure periods
of unemployment with fewer mental and physical symptoms, and even have lower cholesterol levels, than unem-
ployed men lacking such support.

So, as we noted earlier, our personal vicissitudes are ines-
capably tied to those around us. When we suffer, we need to
be comforted and to comfort others; when disabled, we need
protection and are needed to protect others; when dying, we
need others to help us and our help is needed by them.
There is no territory of splendid seclusion where we can live
untouched by other people and immune to the physical environment, where we can become so physically fit that we

will be invulnerable and indominable. There is no sanctuary where people age more slowly, where we are not subject to other people's fallibility, where human beings don't cry out for other human beings when they are in pain. To ameliorate our dis-ease, we must cultivate the social support which we all require; we must nurture the activities and institutions which build cohesion.

Dispelling Solitude

On a personal level, when it comes to health concerns, a burden shared is a burden made lighter. You need someone to comb your hair when you feel too sick to do it, to read aloud to you or hold your hand, to pass the afternoon sitting beside your bed. Listening is one way we can share the burden, of dispelling the unhealthy effects of solitude. We have almost all had the opportunity, at one time or another, to help someone who was sick just by letting him tell his tale. Listening, with as much respect, compassion, and courage as we can muster, lessens the sick person's fears and discomfort.

Listening can do more than deepen supportive personal relationships, though that alone is reason enough for it. It can also be part of an active coping process. This is because people often come up with the solutions to their own problems if allowed to talk them out. People somehow learn to bear even the most awful situations, if we stand by them as they grope toward the answers they need, if we but accompany them on their journey to make peace with their fears and their losses.

Attentive, empathic listening has this effect because it helps the speaker to express himself and in so doing he begins to formulate ideas which have lain inchoate until now. If the listener is good, something new is born in this process of telling, because the speaker does more than merely repeat aloud what he has already thought out and "whispered over to himself"; expression creates.[15] As Cabot and Dicks wrote fifty years ago in a book on caring for patients, "Proper listening builds in the patient more power to meet and to answer . . . questions about the life he has lived and about the future ahead of him. It has been our experience again and again to listen while a patient described his problems, to be stumped by them and appalled at our own failure, and prudently to keep silence and make no answer till that very silence drew the patient on to say more than he started to say. Soon he begins answering himself better than we could have answered him. Before the end of the visit we have often seen him cheered and enlightened, not by anything we have said but by what our silent interest has led him to discover for himself."[16]

But beyond any concrete solutions that grow out of intimate dialogue, there is human consolation and sharing. Above the entrance to Presbyterian Hospital in New York City is carved the ancient quote: "It is the physician's privilege to cure rarely, to alleviate sometimes, but to comfort always." There really are times in life when all we can do is huddle together for comfort in the bottom of the boat. That may be, after all, exactly what we need most just now.

Illness Will Always Be with Us

And so the paradox recurs: we can't feel healthier or more physically secure until we acknowledge the very vulnerability and mortality we are trying so hard to deny. To subdue our fears of disease and ill health, we must confront them and acknowledge their basis in reality: some afflictions are incurable, some ailments unavoidable. The dream of eradicating impairment and abolishing infirmity will go unrealized. There are two unhappy truths: first, aging and suffering and sickness are inherent and inextricable aspects of life; and second, medical science and medical care have their limits. The bad news is that in large measure we do not control our health: the personal control of health is substantially limited by heredity, environment, culture, and chance. But the good news is that if we accept this, we will be better able to enjoy the good health we do have.

The belief that we shouldn't have to fall ill or endure pain makes these states seem worse when they do overtake us. We would do better to accept our colds and our dandruff and our sunburn, or some new ailments in their stead, rather than agonizing over them and treating each as if it were worthy of great attention. We will find our afflictions, both serious and trivial, less excruciating when we accept them as a part of life rather than regarding them as something unnecessary that we shouldn't have to put up with. It is impossible to feel hardy and vital when we pay attention to every twinge or wrinkle. We will feel more robust if we tolerate aging gracefully, rather than trying to postpone it with face-lifts and creams to camouflage "age spots." The same thing is true for society as a whole: a realistic sense of well-being requires that we acknowledge the limits to our ability to improve human health. The fact is that while we can journey to the moon and replace a human heart with a pump, we cannot stop hiccoughing or prevent nearsightedness.

There are situations in life, and illness is sometimes one of them, in which we can't feel better until we accept the fact that we won't get better. It is only then, in adapting to obstacles and frailties, that we can really plumb our own strength and resiliency and resourcefulness. Only when the suffering patient realizes that he is going to have to live with his afflictions does he begin to cope with them. As long as the patient expects to be relieved of his malady, he is detained from the business of learning to minimize it and make the best of his situation. And it is this coping process that ultimately makes discomfort tolerable. As long as the patient remains dedicated to searching for the Holy Grail—the one doctor who can cure him, or the miracle drug that will render his illness nothing more than a bad memory—he will not be able to tolerate his symptoms or overlook them. This is as true of the hypochondriac as it is of the common-cold sufferer and the cancer victim.

A clinical example illustrates this. Patty Baldwin was a paralegal who developed Raynaud's disease in her late twenties. This is a disease of the blood vessels that results in painful spasms in the hands, particularly in cold weather. Though no cure exists, patients can be helped with medications, biofeedback, and meticulous self-care (for example, wearing especially warm mittens and avoiding exposure to the cold). But Patty believed that somewhere there must be a cure for her problem. She felt cheated and dissatisfied, and finding a cure became a personal crusade. She sought out one specialist after another and read everything she could find on the subject. She thought continuously about her plight. Feeling as she did, the periodic attacks of pain seemed agonizing. She began arriving later and later for work on winter mornings because she was waiting for the weather to warm up. Soon, she found herself in almost constant pain.

Eventually, Patty's physician helped her to face the reality that she had an incurable disease, one which is lifelong and poorly understood. Only then did she begin putting her energies into living with it rather than getting rid of it. She curtailed her use of pain relievers, realizing that no matter how much she took, she would always have some discomfort. She accepted a referral for biofeedback therapy that she had previously refused. Though her painful attacks continued, Patty gradually felt less tormented by her symptoms, was less disabled by them (she began, for example, to arrive at work on time again), and was less preoccupied with her illness. Paradoxically, Patty got better once she accepted the fact that she wasn't going to get better.

Many gravely ill people function better, and are more contented and happy, than healthy hypochondriacs. Why? Because they have accepted the reality of their situation, and having done so they set out to make the best of it. They know there is nothing to be gained from studying every ache, since it won't make things any better. For hypochondriacs, on the other hand, each symptom deserves attention because they still believe it is curable, because it is an additional clue in a diagnostic mystery they still think can be solved. People who can accept the awful truth that they have a chronic disease may thus experience less dis-ease than healthy hypochondriacs who are engrossed in their difficulties and wrapped up in their fears. It *is* possible to accept ill health with some degree of equanimity. People can learn to live amazingly well without something they treasured, once they know with absolute certainty and finality in their hearts that they will never have it; but they can't adapt to a loss when they imagine that there is still a remote chance of getting back what they have lost. We are more tormented by disappointments and limitations when we harbor the fantasy that one day the laws of nature might be evaded, or the clock turned back, or human nature suspended, then when we let the truth sink in. Only then can we mourn our loss and let it go, only then can we make peace with what has happened to us.

It is not that we should abandon the pursuit of health. We should not stop seeking healthier lifestyles, or curtail our biomedical research, or obtain less medical care. Nor should we ignore the problems of pollution or stress or diet, or disregard the importance of the psyche in health. But we must place them in perspective and keep a sense of proportion about our quest. We need not alter our course so much as appreciate that we may not travel as fast or as far along it as we thought. Such a sense of proportion will protect us from finding our medical advances too meager when compared with our efforts and our expectations. Without this, our quest may become counterproductive, as expectations outstrip accomplishments, and advances seem unsatisfactory and inadequate.

Forging Strength out of Illness

To become truly human, to throw oneself fully into life, is to know its injuries and its dangers. Ultimately, it is the specter of death that casts life into high relief and helps us to relish and appreciate it. Goethe observed that only through the acceptance of death can man reap all there is in life; without that ultimate acknowledgment of man's condition, his life is diminished and less significant.[17] Freud made a similar point when he observed that a knowledge of the impermanence of our love objects makes us love them more. Abiding commitments, deep love, and a full appreciation of life are frightening because they bring us face to face with our own mortality, with the transience and fragility of all life. But they also become that much more valuable in this light. To contemplate the loss of a loved one through accident or disease is to appreciate him all the more; to dedicate yourself to accomplishing some life's work means acknowledging that you may not be given the time to complete it; to appreciate the natural world is to realize the insignificance of human life in the larger scheme of things. One of the ironies of the human experience is that we sometimes have to face illness or injury or even the possibility of death in order to discover a sense of purpose and to decide how best to live a rewarding life. An awareness of life's tenuousness enriches the pleasure and the meaning we find in it.

Losses are an inescapable part of life: the loss of youth, the loss of bodily vigor and bodily performance, the loss of independence, the death of loved ones. To deny these losses is to deny our humanity. We can't live full lives without being wounded by the losses we've sustained along the way. But wounds heal, if we let them, and though a scar remains, reminding us that what we lost was an important part of us, scars don't hurt. We ought not be so afraid of facing our physical limitations and losses, for as the psychoanalyst Elvin Semrad said, "People grow only around sadness; it's strange to be arranged that way, but that's the way it seems to be."[18]

Recently a fifty-five-year-old chest surgeon wrote eloquently of his five-year experience with metastatic lung cancer.[19] He expresses an attitude about death, a peace and a resignation, that are increasingly rare. He has had to curtail his work schedule, face his professional colleagues, reexamine his religious beliefs, and learn how to gradually relinquish life. He describes his search for meaning in what life he has left and his growing appreciation of nature, gardening, personal relationships, and family. He speaks of death with an acceptance devoid of bitterness, loss of control, or defeat. "I have ceased to feel that death is a dreadful something that I need to fear. Instead, it will ultimately appear as a peaceful act of letting go when the time comes and I am ready. We are all dying; the difference between persons is only in the length and quality of the time that is left. Death ceases to be the failure; the failure is in not being willing to make the effort to grow and change. . . . Life becomes a great river that will flow no matter what I do. I can flow with it and live in peace, or I can slip back into old patterns and live in despair, fighting against the current. The river does not care. It only makes a difference to me and to those around me. The choice is mine."

He notes that his preparations to die, such as making out his will and arranging to provide for his family, have "been associated not with a sense of impending doom or imminent death but with a sense that making these arrangements now frees me from future concern. . . . I am very grateful just to be alive. I am very glad to have been permitted to learn to live with, rather than simply die from, my cancer. . . . When my days are no longer nourishing and good, I hope that I can simply let go and allow myself to rest in peace. . . . In each of the last three autumns, I have wondered whether to plant the tulip and daffodil bulbs for the spring bloom or not to bother. Now, again this past spring, a glory of living color rewarded me, and once again I have planted for next spring's blooming."

People who feel they have truly lived life are less afraid of dying, of being cheated by illness. The more we feel that we are getting what we want out of life, the less we worry about our bodies giving out on us. As we come to value the journey more than the destination, we can appreciate where we are rather than worrying whether we have the strength and endurance to get farther ahead. Our insatiable appetite for medical care and preventive health measures, this perpetual need for more—to survive at all costs, to live a day longer, to sculpt a flawless appearance, to be perfectly fit—stems from a failure to fully experience what we do have. And if we can learn to get more out of our work and our relationships, to experience a fuller emotional life, if we can cultivate the ability to play and to appreciate nature, we will feel less cheated, less desperate for a slimmer waistline and more medical information, less afraid of getting sick.

A mature and realistic appreciation of our impermanence and our vulnerability does not result in hopelessness but in a quiet pride, in a delight with what life offers, and in the strength to face illness and suffering. It is in this crucible of coping with adversity that a true sense of physical well-being can be forged. We should aim to live as successfully as possible with what we have, rather than trying to avoid what can't be avoided, to overcome what can't be overcome, to ignore what ultimately can't be ignored. For in the final analysis, it is sounder to believe that we can cope with illness should it befall us than to believe we can escape it. In believing that we can evade disease, avoid disability, escape the ravages of old age, and even postpone death itself, we fail to see and to appreciate our remarkable capacity to persevere and survive in spite of these inevitabilities; we fail to build confidence in our abilities to adapt and to cope; we miss the opportunity to develop a sense of ourselves as strong enough to endure misfortune when it does occur. We learn about our strength and vitality by getting the most out of what we have and what is possible, given our particular age, our physical capacities, our medical status. We can learn to cope with and live with illness, as well as learning to cure it and prevent it, and the former is every bit as important as the latter.

Notes

CHAPTER ONE

1. Beeson, P. B. "One hundred years of American internal medicine." *Annals of Internal Medicine* 105 (1986): 436–444.
2. Shorter, E. *Bedside Manners*. (New York: Simon and Schuster, 1985), pp. 180–183.
3. Ibid., p. 133; see also Rosenberg, C. E. "What it was like to be sick in 1884." *American Heritage* 35 (October–November 1984): 23–31.
4. Belloc, N. B., and Breslow, L. "Relationship of physical health status and health practices." *Preventive Medicine* 1 (1972): 409–421.
5. Fuchs, V. *Who Shall Live? Economics and Social Choice*. (New York: Basic Books, 1974), p. 52–55.
6. Goldman, L., and Cook, E. F.: "Decline in ischemic heart disease mortality." *Annals of Internal Medicine* 101 (1984): 825–836.
7. *Health, United States, 1985*. National Center for Health Statistics. (Washington, DC: National Center for Health Statistics, Public Health Service, USDHHS, 1985. DHHS Pub. No. 86–1232), p. 40.
8. Rogers, D. E., and Blendon, R. J. "The changing American health scene." *Journal of the American Medical Association* 237 (1977): 1710–1714. See also *Health, United States, 1985, p. 40*.
9. *Health, United States, 1985, p. 38*.
10. Rogers, D. E., and Blendon, R. J. "The changing American health scene," pp. 1710–1714.
11. *Health, United States, 1985*, p. 41.
12. Miller, J. *The Body in Question*. (New York: Vintage Books, 1982), pp. 106–141.
13. Thomas, L. *The Lives of a Cell*. (New York: Bantam Books, 1975), p. 100.

CHAPTER TWO

1. Small, G. W., and Nicholi, A. M. "Mass hysteria among schoolchildren." *Archives of General Psychiatry* 39 (1982): 721–724.

2. Dunnell, K., and Cartwright, A. *Medicine Takers, Prescribers, and Hoarders.* (London: Routledge and Kegan Paul, 1972); see also Hanney, D. R. *The Symptom Iceberg: A Study of Community Health.* (London: Routledge and Kegan Paul, 1979); and Wadsworth, M. E. J., Butterfield, W. J. H., and Blaney, R. *Health and Sickness: The Choice of Treatment.* (London: Tavistock, 1972).

3. Hanney, *The Symptom Iceberg;* see also Wadsworth et al., *Health and Sickness.*

4. Belloc, N. B., Breslow, L., and Hochstein, J. R. "Measurement of physical health in a general population survey." *American Journal of Epidemiology* 93 (1971): 328–336.

5. Antonovsky, A. *Health, Stress, and Coping.* (San Francisco: Jossey-Bass, 1980); see also Zola, I. K. "The omnipresence of illness." *Journal of the Netherlands College of General Practitioners* 16 (1973): 427–430.

6. Beecher, H. K. "Relationship of significance of wound to pain experienced." *Journal of the American Medical Association* 161 (1956): 1609–1613.

7. Ibid., pp. 1609, 1611.

8. Pennebaker, J. W., and Skelton, J. A. "Selective monitoring of bodily sensations." *Journal of Personality and Social Psychology* 41 (1981): 213–223.

9. Wheeler, E. O., Williamson, C. R., and Cohen, M. E. "Heart scare, heart surveys, and iatrogenic heart disease." *Journal of the American Medical Association* 167 (1958): 1096–1102.

10. Nisbett, R. E., and Schachter, S. "Cognitive manipulation of pain." *Journal of Experimental and Social Psychology* 2 (1966): 227–236.

11. Storms, M. D., and Nisbett, R. E. "Insomnia and the attribution process." *Journal of Personality and Social Psychology* 16 (1970): 319–328.

12. Pennebaker, J. W. *The Psychology of Physical Symptoms.* (New York: Springer-Verlag, 1982).

13. Wicklund, R. "Objective Self-Awareness." In *Advances in Experimental Social Psychology,* vol. 8, ed. L. Berkowitz. (New York: Academic Press, 1975), pp. 233–275.

14. Pennebaker, J. W. "Perceptual and environmental determinants of coughing." *Basic and Applied Social Psychology* 1 (1980): 83–91.

15. Levine, J. D., Gordon, N. C., Smith, R., and Fields, H. L. "Post-operative pain: Effect of extent of injury and attention." *Brain Research* 234 (1982): 500–504.

16. Pennebaker, J. W. *The Psychology of Physical Symptoms,* p. 25.

17. Ibid., pp. 135–139; see also Mechanic, D. "Development of psychological distress among young adults." *Archives of General Psychiatry* 36 (1979): 1233–1239.

CHAPTER THREE

1. Peterson, W. L., Sturdevant, R. A. L., Frankl, H. D., et al. "Healing of duodenal ulcer with an antacid regimen." *New England Journal of Medicine* 297 (1977): 341–345.

2. Petrie, A. *Individuality in Pain and Suffering,* 2d edition. (Chicago: University of Chicago Press, 1978).

3. Pennebaker, J. W. *The Psychology of Physical Symptoms.* (New York: Springer-Verlag, 1982), pp. 5–9.

4. Sternbach, R. A., and Tursky, B. "Ethnic differences among housewives in psychophysical and skin potential responses to electric shock." *Psychophysiology* 1 (1965): 241–246; Tursky, B., and Sternbach, R. A. "Further physiological correlates of ethnic differences in responses to shock." *Psychophysiology* 4 (1967): 67–74; Weisenberg, M. "Pain and pain control." *Psychology Bulletin* 84 (1977): 1008–1044.

5. Zola, I. K. "Culture and symptoms—an analysis of patients' presenting complaints." *American Sociological Review* 31 (1966): 615–630.

6. Zborowski, M. *People in Pain.* (San Francisco: Jossey-Bass, 1969).

7. ———. "Cultural components in response to pain." *Journal of Social Issues* 8 (1952): 16–30.

8. Campbell, A. *The Sense of Well-Being in America.* (New York: McGraw-Hill, 1981), p. 208.

9. Mechanic, D. "The experience and expression of distress: The study of illness behavior and medical utilization." *Handbook of Health, Health Care, and the Health Professions,* ed. D. Mechanic. (New York: Free Press, 1983), p. 596.

10. Ibid.

11. Pennebaker, J. W. *The Psychology of Physical Symptoms,* p. 136.

12. Ibid., page 137.

13. Rodin, J. "Something about convalescent home residents and control and mortality rates." *Science* 233 (1986): 1271–1276.

14. Campbell, A. *The Sense of Well-Being in America,* pp. 214–216.

15. Hunter, R. C. A., Lohrenz, J. G., and Schwartzman, A. E. "Nosophobia and hypochondriasis in medical students." *Journal of Nervous and Mental Disorders* 139 (1964): 147–152.

16. Proust, M. *À la recherche du temps perdu. Vol. 11: Le Côté de Guermantes.* (Paris: Gallimard, 1920–21), p. 153.

17. Ehrlich, R. *The Healthy Hypochondriac: Recognizing, Understanding, and Living with Anxiety About Our Health.* (Philadelphia: Saunders Press, 1980), pp. 97, 186.

18. Carlson, E. T. "Hypochondriasis." *International Journal of Psychiatry* 2 (1966): 676–679.

CHAPTER FOUR

1. Ehrlich, R. *The Healthy Hypochondriac: Recognizing, Understanding, and Living with Anxieties About Our Health.* (Philadelphia: Saunders Press, 1980), p. 180.

2. Rako, S., and Mazer, H. *Semrad: The Heart of a Therapist.* (New York: Jason Aronson, 1980), pp. 175–176.

3. Brown, H. N., Vaillant, G. E. "Hypochondriasis." *Archives of Internal Medicine* 141 (1981): 723–726.

4. Ehrlich, R. *The Healthy Hypochondriac,* p. 75.

5. Minuchin, L., Rosman, B. L., and Baker, L. *Psychosomatic Families.* (Cambridge: Harvard University Press, 1978), p. 32.

6. Ibid., no specific page.

7. Mechanic, D. "Development of psychological distress among young adults." *Archives of General Psychiatry* 36 (1979): 1233–1239.

8. Kleinman, A. "Neurasthenia and depression: A study of somatization and culture in China." *Culture, Medicine and Psychiatry* 6 (1982): 117–190.

9. Leff, J. P. "Culture and the differentiation of emotional states." *British Journal of Psychiatry* 123 (1973): 299–306.

CHAPTER FIVE

1. Rubenstein, C. "Wellness is all. A report on *Psychology Today's* survey of beliefs about health." *Psychology Today* (October 1982): 28–37.

2. Harris, L. *Inside America.* (New York: Vintage Books, 1987), p. 40.

3. Crawford, R. "A cultural account of 'health': Control, release, and the social body." In *Contemporary Issues in Health, Medicine, and Social Policy,* ed. J. B. McKinlay. (New York: Tavistock, 1984), pp. 60–103. Some evidence even suggests that the pursuit of the healthy lifestyle is more prevalent among the working classes, for example, a poll by Yankelovich, Skelly, and White revealed that while 60 percent of Harvard and Stanford alumni regard "staying in good shape" as very important, this figure is lower than the 80 percent of the general population who answered this positively. Skelly, F. "To the beat of a different drum." *Harvard Magazine* (March–April 1986): pp. 21–27.

4. Gurin, J. "The us generation." *American Health* (October 1985), pp. 40–41.

5. Wallis, C. "One miracle, many doubts." *Time* (December 10, 1984): p. 72.

6. ———. "Of television and transplants." *Time* (June 23, 1986): p. 68.

7. Clark, M. "Search for a cure." *Newsweek* (December 16, 1985), pp. 60–65.

8. Toufexis, A. "Shake a leg, Mrs. Plushbottom." *Time* (June 2, 1986), pp. 78–80.

9. Sigerist, H. E. *On the Sociology of Medicine.* (New York: MD Publications, 1960), pp. 9–22.

10. Ibid.

11. Ibid.

12. Ibid.

13. Institute of Medicine, Committee on Pain, Disability, and Chronic Illness Behavior. *Pain and Disability,* eds M. Osterweis, A. Kleinman, and D. Mechanic. (Washington, DC: National Academy Press, 1987).

14. Katon, W., Ries, R. K., and Kleinman, A. "The prevalence of somatization in primary care." *Comprehensive Psychiatry* 25 (1984): 208–215.

15. Yelin, E., Nevitt, M., Epstein, W. "Toward an epidemiology of work disability." *Milbank Memorial Fund Quarterly* 58 (1980): 386–415.

16. Stone, D. A. "Diagnosis and the dole: The function of illness in American distributive politics." *Journal of Health Politics, Policy and Law* 4 (1979): 507–521.

17. Institute of Medicine, Committee on Pain, Disability, and Chronic Illness Behavior. *Pain and Disability.*

18. Katon, W., Ries, R. K., and Kleinman, A. "The prevalence of somatization in primary care."

19. Stone, D. A. "Diagnosis and the dole," pp. 507–521.

20. Blumberg, B. S., Millman, I., and London, W. T. "Ted Slavin's blood and the development of the HBV vaccine." *New England Journal of Medicine* 312 (1985): 189.

21. Harris, L. *Inside America,* p. 13.

22. Gillick, M. R. "Health promotion, jogging, and the pursuit of the moral life." *Journal of Health Politics, Policy and Law* 9 (1984): 369–387; see also Yates, A., Leehey, K., and Shisslak, C. M. "Running: An analogue of anorexia?" *New England Journal of Medicine* 308 (1983): 251–255.

23. Danish, S. J. "Musings about personal competence: The contributions of sport, health, and fitness." *American Journal of Community Psychology* 11 (1983): 221–240.

24. Gillick, M. R. "Health promotion, jogging, and the pursuit of the moral life," p. 374.

25. Koplan, J. P., Siscovick, D. S., and Goldbaum, G. M. "The risks of exercise: A public health view of injuries and hazards." *Public Health Reports* 100 (1985): 189–195.

26. Toufexis, A. "Watch the bouncing body." *Time* (June 30, 1986): p. 74.

27. Cobb, N. "A nation getting into shape." *Boston Globe* (April 1, 1984).

28. Toufexis, A. "Working out in a personal gym." *Time* (February 10, 1986): p. 74; see also Cobb, N. "A nation getting into shape."
29. Cobb, N. "A nation getting into shape."
30. Toufexis, A. "Working out in a personal gym," p. 74.
31. Sabol, B. "Jamie Lee Curtis is a 'perfect' body." *American Health* (May 1985): p. 64.
32. Gillick, M. "Health promotion, jogging, and the pursuit of the moral life," p. 377.
33. Sheehan, G. *Running and Being.* (New York: Simon and Schuster, 1979).
34. Gillick, M. R. "Health promotion, jogging, and the pursuit of the moral life," pp. 379–380.
35. Reed, J. D. "America shapes up." *Time* (November 2, 1981), p. 104.
36. Lipsyte, R. "What price fitness?" *New York Times Magazine* (February 16, 1986), p. 32.
37. Haley, B. *The Healthy Body and Victorian Culture.* (Cambridge: Harvard University Press, 1978), pp. 124–140.
38. Ibid., pp. 253–261.
39. Harris, L. *Inside America,* p. 12.
40. Hall, T. "Steady diet: What Americans eat hasn't changed much despite healthy image." *Wall Street Journal* (September 12, 1985).
41. Burros, M. "Who buys it? The affluent and the aware." *New York Times* (April 2, 1986).
42. Sherman, S. P. "America's new abstinence." *Fortune* (March 18, 1985): 20–23.
43. "Health facts: A baker's dozen." *New York Times Magazine,* pt. 2 (September 28, 1986): pp. 32–33.
44. "Implications of vitamin use." *FDA Drug Bulletin* 13 (1983): 27–28.
45. Katz, S. "Getting sick on vitamins." *Newsweek* (May 19, 1986), p. 80.
46. Beck, A. "Extra calcium: Who needs it?" *Boston Globe* (February 18, 1987).
47. Burros, M. "Who buys it?"
48. Haas, R. *Eat to Succeed.* (New York: Rawson Associates, 1986), dust jacket.
49. Berger, S. *Doctor Berger's Immune Power Diet.* (New York: New American Library, 1985), national advertisement.
50. Toufexis, A. "Dieting: The losing game." *Time* (January 20, 1986): 54.
51. Garner, D. M., Garfinkel, P. E., and Olmsted, M. P. "An overview of sociocultural factors in the development of anorexia nervosa." In *Anorexia Nervosa: Recent Developments in Research,* ed. L. Padraig and E. Darby. (New York: A. R. Liss, 1983), p. 70.
52. Kleinfield, N. R. "The ever-fatter business of thinness." *New York*

Times (September 7, 1986); see also Kanner, B. "Chubby Checkers." *New York Times* (February 18, 1985).

53. Kleinfield, N. R. "The ever-fatter business of thinness."
54. Schwartz, D. M., Thompson, M. G., and Johnson, C. L. "Anorexia nervosa and bulimia: The socio-cultural context." *International Journal of Eating Disorders* 1 (1981–82); 20–36.
55. Sheraton, M. "Figures can't lie but . . ." *Time* (January 20, 1986), p. 62.
56. Ibid.
57. Gerbner, G., Morgan, M., and Signorielli, N. "Programming health portrayals: What viewers see, say, and do." In *Television and Behavior,* vol. 2, ed. D. Pearl, L. Bouthilet, and J. Lazar. (Washington, DC: USDHEW, Publication # ADM 82-1196), pp. 291–307.
58. Ibid.
59. Stoeckle, J. D. "Medical advice books: The search for the healthy body." *Social Science and Medicine* 18 (1984): 707–712.
60. Toufexis, A. "The shape of the nation." *Time* (October 7, 1985), p. 60.
61. *The World Almanac 1966.* (New York: New York World–Telegram Corp., 1966), p. 512.
62. Bechtel, S. "Affordable American health spas." *Prevention* (May 1985), p. 126.
63. Ginzberg, E. A hard look at cost containment. *New England Journal of Medicine* 316 (1987): 1151–1154.
64. Ibid.
65. *Information Please Almanac,* 38th ed. (Boston: Houghton Mifflin Company, 1985).
66. Ginzberg E.: A hard look at cost containment, pp. 1151–1154.
67. Fein, R. "Social and economic attitudes shaping American health policy." *Milbank Memorial Fund Quarterly* 58 (1980): 358.
68. Levey, S., and Hesse, D. D. "Bottom-line Health Care." *New England Journal of Medicine* 312 (1985): 644–647.
69. *Quackery: A $10 Billion Scandal.* Report of the Select Committee on Aging, House of Representatives. (Washington, DC: United States Government Printing Office, Publication #98-435, 1984), p. 3.
70. Ibid.
71. Conrad, P. "Implications of changing social policy for the medicalization of deviance." *Contemporary Crises* 4 (1980): 195–205.
72. Greenwald, J. "Those sky-high health costs." *Time* (July 12, 1982), p. 54.
73. Fein, R. "Social and economic attitudes shaping American health policy."
74. Thurow, L. C. "Medicine versus economics." *New England Journal of Medicine* 313 (1985): 611–614.

75. Freidson, E. Profession of Medicine. (New York: Dodd, Mead, 1970), pp. 245–246.
76. Crawford, R. "Healthism and the medicalization of everyday life." *International Journal of Health Services* 10 (1980): 365–388.
77. Ibid.
78. Ibid., pp. 380–381.
79. Ibid., p. 380.
80. Becker, M. H. "The tyranny of health promotion." *Public Health Review* 14 (1986): 20.

CHAPTER SIX

1. *Health, United States, 1985.* (Washington, DC: National Center for Health Statistics, USDHHS, 1985), DHHS Pub. No. 86-1232, p. 82.
2. Stoeckle, J. D., and White, G. A. *Plain Pictures of Plain Doctoring.* (Boston: MIT Press, 1985), p. 54.
3. Shorter, E. *Bedside Manners.* (New York: Simon and Schuster, 1985), p. 110.
4. Ibid., pp. 113–114.
5. Ibid., p. 214.
6. Ibid.
7. Barker, L. R. "Distinctive Characteristics of Ambulatory Medicine." In *Principles of Ambulatory Medicine,* ed. L. R. Barker, J. R. Burton, P. D. Zieve. (Baltimore: Williams and Wilkins, 1982), pp. 1–15.
8. Kass, L. "Regarding the end of medicine and the pursuit of health." *The Public Interest* 40 (1975): 11–42, p. 11.
9. Conrad, P. "Implications of changing social policy for the medicalization of deviance." *Contemporary Crises* 4 (1980): 195–205.
10. Friedson, E. *Profession of Medicine.* (New York: Dodd, Mead, 1970), p. 247.
11. Zola, I. K. "Medicine as an institution of social control." *Sociological Review* 20 (1972: 487–504); see also ———. "The concept of trouble and sources of medical assistance: To whom one can turn, with what, and why." *Social Science and Medicine* 6 (1972): 673–679.
12. Conrad, P., and Schneider, J. W. *Deviance and Medicalization.* (St. Louis, MO: E. V. Mosby, 1980), pp. 73–109.
13. Conrad, P. "Implications of changing social policy for the medicalization of deviance," pp. 195–205.
14. Conrad, P., and Schneider, J. W. *Deviance and Medicalization,* pp. 73–109.
15. Ibid., pp. 110–144.
16. Ibid.
17. Ibid., pp. 215–224.
18. Ibid., pp. 161–170.

19. Ibid.

20. Ibid., pp. 155–160.

21. Schechter, N. L. "The baby and the bathwater: Hyperactivity and the medicalization of child rearing." *Perspectives in Biology and Medicine* 25 (1982): 406–416.

22. Ibid.

23. Smilgis, M. "Snip, suction, stretch and truss." *Time* (September 14, 1987): 70.

24. Adler, J. "New bodies for sale." *Newsweek* (May 27, 1985): 64.

25. Ibid.

26. Giddon, D. B. "Through the looking glasses of physicians, dentists, and patients." *Perspectives in Biology and Medicine* 26 (1983): 451–458.

27. Garner, D. M., Garfinkel, P. E., and Olmsted, M. P. "An Overview of Sociocultural Factors in the Development of Anorexia Nervosa." In *Anorexia Nervosa: Recent Developments in Research,* ed. L. Padraig and E. Darby. (New York: A. R. Liss, 1983), pp. 65–82.

28. Garner, D. M., Garfinkel, P. E., Schwartz, D., and Thompson, M. "Cultural expectations of thinness in women." *Psychological Reports* 47 (1980): 483–491.

29. Atkinson, H. *Women and Fatigue.* (New York: G. P. Putnam's Sons, 1986), advertisement.

30. Seligmann, J.: "Malaise of the '80s: The puzzling and debilitating Epstein-Barr virus." *Newsweek* (October 27, 1986): 105–106.

31. *New York Times Magazine,* Part II, "The Good Health Magazine" (September 28, 1986): advertisement for Schiff.

32. Ford, C. V. *The Somatizing Disorders.* (New York: Elsevier Biomedical, 1983), pp. 18–19; Ford, C. V., Bray, G. A., and Swerdloff, R. S. "A psychiatric study of patients referred with a diagnosis of hypoglycemia." *American Journal of Psychiatry* 133 (1976): 290–294.

33. Winston, B. V. "Psychologists cite fans' reactions to Sox loss." *Boston Globe* (October 29, 1986).

34. Our therapeutic zeal has even filtered down to children's literature. New books for four-to-seven-year-olds focus on their worries, seeking to cure or reassure them by bringing their difficulties into the open, from fears of being bullied in school to sibling rivalry at home, from the difficulties of having a single parent to having a bedroom that is too small. Morrison, B. "The age of anxiety." *Times Literary Supplement* (February 14, 1986), p. 174.

35. Relman, A. S. "The new medical-industrial complex." *New England Journal of Medicine* 303 (1980): 963–970.

36. Reice, S. "The anti-aging lifestyle." *Ladies Home Journal* (September 1984), p. 115.

37. Relman, A. S. Personal communication.
38. "The new medical-industrial complex," pp. 933–970.
39. Alper, P. A. "Medical practice in the competitive market." *New England Journal of Medicine* 316 (1987): 337–339.
40. Gray, J. "The selling of medicine." *Medical Economics* (January 20, 1986), p. 180.
41. Koepp, S. "Hospitals learn the hard sell." *Time* (January 12, 1987), p. 56.
42. Ibid.
43. Williams, W. "Cashing in on fitness foods." *New York Times* (November 4, 1984).
44. Sapolsky, H. M. "The politics of product controversies." In *Consuming Fears,* ed. H. M. Sapolsky. (New York: Basic Books, 1986), pp. 182–201.
45. Greer, W. M. "Health fairs move into mainstream." *New York Times* (April 2, 1986).
46. Illich, I. *Medical Nemesis.* (New York: Pantheon Books, 1976), pp. 111–116.
47. Ibid., see also Powles, J. "On the limitations of modern medicine." *Science, Medicine and Man* 1 (1973): 1–30.
48. Starr, P. *The Social Transformation of American Medicine.* (New York: Basic Books, 1982), pp. 35–37.
49. Ibid.
50. Hanney, D. R. *The Symptom Iceberg: A Study of Community Health.* (London: Routledge and Kegan Paul, 1979), p. 145.
51. Hareven, T. K. "American families in transition: Historical perspectives on change." In *Normal Family Processes,* ed. F. Walsh. (New York: The Guilford Press, 1982), pp. 446–466.
52. Shorter, E. *Bedside Manners,* pp. 217–218.
53. Starr, P. *The Social Transformation of American Medicine,* pp. 73–75; see also Hareven, T. K. "American families in transition, pp. 446–466.
54. Macdonald, L. A., Sackett, D. L., Haynes, R. B., and Taylor, D. W. "Labelling and hypertension: A review of the behavioral and psychological consequences." *Journal of Chronic Disease* 37 (1984): 933–942.

CHAPTER SEVEN

1. Bauman, E. "Introduction to holistic health." In *The Holistic Health Handbook,* ed. Berkeley Holistic Health Center. (Berkeley, CA: And/Or Press, 1978), p. 19.
2. Kinderlehrer, J. "How to save yourself from a dangerous cancer." *Prevention* (May 1985): pp. 110, 112.

3. Crawford, R. "A cultural account of 'health': Control, release and the social body." In *Contemporary Issues in Health, Medicine, and Social Policy,* ed. J. B. McKinlay. (New York: Tavistock Publications, 1984), pp. 60–103.

4. Ibid.

5. Bennett, W., and Gurin, J. *The Dieter's Dilemma: Eating Less and Weighing More.* (New York: Basic Books, 1982), pp. 274–278; see also Crawford, R. "A cultural account of 'health.'"

6. Crawford, R. "A cultural account of 'health.'"

7. Garner, D. M., Garfinkel, P. E., and Olmsted, M. P. "An overview of sociocultural factors in the development of anorexia nervosa." In *Anorexia Nervosa: Recent Developments in Research,* ed. L. Padraig and E. Darby. (New York: A. R. Liss, 1983), pp. 65–82.

8. Ibid.

9. Crawford, R: "A cultural account of 'health.'"

10. Ibid.

11. Ibid., p. 66.

12. Fuchs, V. R. *How We Live.* (Cambridge: Harvard University Press, 1983), pp. 107–108.

13. Shorter, E. *Bedside Manners.* (New York: Simon and Schuster, 1985), p. 121.

14. "Private practice." *Time* (November 25, 1985), p. 85.

15. Ibid.

16. Ibid.

17. Levin, L. S., and Idler, E. L. "Self-care in health." *Annual Review of Public Health* 4 (1983): 181–201.

18. Morantz, R. M. "Nineteenth-century health reform and women: A program for self-help." In *Medicine Without Doctors: Home Health Care in American History,* eds. G. B. Risse, R. L. Numbers, and J. W. Leavitt. (New York: Science History Publishers, 1977), pp. 73–93; see also Risse, G. B., Numbers, R. L., and Leavitt, J. W. *Medicine without Doctors: Home Health Care in American History.* (New York: Science History Publishing, 1977); Whorton, J. C. *Crusaders for Fitness.* (Princeton, NJ: Princeton University Press, 1982).

19. Whorton, J. C. *Crusaders for Fitness;* see also Risse et al., *Medicine without Doctors;* Morantz, "Nineteenth-century health reform and women"; and Starr, P. *The Social Transformation of American Medicine.* (New York: Basic Books, 1982), pp. 32–37.

20. Raver, A. "A trip through the whole health catalog." *Boston Magazine* (December 1985), p. 212.

21. Sontag, S. *Illness as Metaphor.* (New York: Vintage Books, 1979), pp. 54–56.

22. Cassileth, B. R., Lusk, E. J., Miller, D. S., et al. "Psychosocial corre-

lates of survival in advanced malignant disease." *New England Journal of Medicine* 312 (1985): 1551–1556.

23. Angell, M. "Disease as a reflection of the psyche." *New England Journal of Medicine* 312 (1985): 1570–1572.

24. Goleman, D. "Debate intensifies on attitude and health." *New York Times* (October 29, 1985).

25. Muramoto, N. *Healing Ourselves.* (New York: Avon Books, 1973), p. 116.

26. Ardell, D. *High Level Wellness: An Alternative to Doctors, Drugs, and Disease.* (Emmaus, PA: Rodale Press, 1977), p. 2.

27. Jaroff, L. "Can attitudes affect cancer?" *Time* (June 24, 1985), p. 69.

28. Harris, L. *Inside America.* (New York: Vintage Books, 1987), p. 8.

29. Wallis, C. "Stress: Can we cope?" *Time* (June 6, 1983), p. 49.

30. Harris, L. *Inside America,* p. 9.

31. Wallis, "Stress: Can we cope?," p. 48.

32. Rubenstein, C. "Wellness is all." *Psychology Today* (October 1982), p. 28.

33. Sutton, R. *Body Worry.* (New York: Viking, 1987).

34. Toufexis, A. "The rebuilding of Remar Sutton." *Time* (April 6, 1987), p. 72.

35. Duka, J. "Looking good." *New York Times Magazine,* Part 2 (March 3, 1985), p. 154.

36. Smilgis, M. "Snip, suction, stretch and truss." *Time* (September 14, 1987), p. 70.

37. Banner, L. W. *American Beauty.* (New York: Alfred A. Knopf, 1983), pp. 201–205.

38. Ibid., pp. 213–214.

39. Weir, J. "Computing skin care." *New York Times Magazine* (December 9, 1984), pp. 139–144.

40. Toufexis, A. "New rub for the skin game." *Time* (March 31, 1986), p. 61.

41. Ibid.

42. Harris, *Inside America,* p. 222.

43. Blendon, R. J., and Altman, D. E. "Public attitudes about health care costs." *New England Journal of Medicine* 311 (1984): 613–616.

44. Ibid.

45. Navarro, V. "Where is the popular magnate?" *New England Journal of Medicine* 307 (1982): 1517–1518.

46. Blendon, R. J., and Altman D. E. "Public attitudes about health care costs."

47. Ibid.

48. Aaron, H. J., and Schwartz, W. B. *The Painful Prescription: Rationing Health Care.* (Washington, DC: The Brookings Institute, 1984).

49. Ibid., pp. 27–76.
50. Ibid., pp. 100–112.
51. Ibid., p. 37.

CHAPTER EIGHT

1. Thomas, L. *The Medusa and the Snail.* (New York: Bantam Books, 1979), pp. 38, 39, 43.
2. Advertisement for Rockport Shoes. *American Health* (October 1985), p. 25.
3. Advertisement for Endometriosis Association. *Time* (February 2, 1987), p. Q1.
4. Zamichow, N. "Chlamydia: Silently devastating." *Boston Globe* (May 26, 1986).
5. Lehman, B. A. "The prostate: Ignore it at your peril." *Boston Globe* (January 12, 1987).
6. "Too much TV linked to obese youngsters." *Boston Globe* (1986).
7. Dietz, W. H., and Gortmaker, S. L. "Do we fatten our children at the television set? Obesity and television viewing in children and adolescents." *Pediatrics* 75 (1985): 807–812.
8. Foley, D. "The chair-sitter's guide to a better bottom half." *Prevention* 37 (May 1985): 92–108 (quotes are from page 92).
9. Reed, J. D. "America shapes up." *Time* (November 2, 1981), p. 94.
10. Starr, D. "The 12-month pregnancy." *American Health* (June 1987), p. 56.
11. "Night Sweats." *Harvard Medical School Health Letter* (October 1986), p. 3.
12. Baker, R. "Observer: The depth of fashion." *New York Times* (November 8, 1986).
13. Ames, B. N. "Dietary carcinogens and anticarcinogens." *Science* 221 (1983): 1256–1264.
14. Thomas, L. *The Medusa and the Snail,* p. 38.
15. Harris, L. *Inside America.* (New York: Vintage Books, 1987), pp. 3–7.
16. Gray, S. H. "Social aspects of body image: Perception of normalcy of weight and affect of college undergraduates." *Perceptual and Motor Skills* 45 (1977): 1035–1040.
17. Lasch, C. *The Culture of Narcissism.* (New York: W. W. Norton and Company, 1978).
18. Ibid., pp. 52–70.
19. Ibid., pp. 3–7.
20. Harris, *Inside America,* p. 5.
21. "Life without bifocals." Advertisement for Varilux, *New Yorker* (March 25, 1985), p. 99.

22. Adler, J. "New bodies for sale." *Newsweek* (May 27, 1985), p. 69.

23. Fisher, D. H. *Growing Old in America*. (New York: Oxford University Press, 1978), pp. 78–101.

24. Banner, L. W. *American Beauty*. (New York: Alfred A. Knopf, 1983), p. 225.

25. Lasch, *The Culture of Narcissism*, pp. 207–217.

26. Davis, F. "How you can look and feel younger." *Ladies Home Journal* (January 1986), p. 62.

27. Lasch, C. *The Culture of Narcissism*, pp. 207–217.

28. Adler, J. "New bodies for sale," pp. 64–69.

29. Fisher, D. H. *Growing Old in America*, p. 134.

30. Ibid., pp. 134, 135.

31. Aharoni, Y. *The No-Risk Society*. (Chatham, NJ: Chatham House Publishers, 1981), p. 53.

32. Fox, R. C. "The evolution of medical uncertainty." *Milbank Memorial Fund Quarterly* 58 (1980): 1–49.

33. "Rising malpractice claims alarm doctors." *Massachusetts General Hospital News* (October 1985), p. 5.

34. Ibid.

35. Murphy, J. "A comeback for whooping cough." *Time* (June 30, 1986), p. 78.

36. Jarvik, M. E. "Necessary risks." *New England Journal of Medicine* 300 (1979): 1330.

37. Aharoni, Y. *The No-Risk Society*, p. 64.

38. Ibid., p. 208.

39. Thomas E. "The new untouchables?" *Time* (September 23, 1985), p. 24.

40. Morrow, Lance. "The start of a plague mentality." *Time* (September 23, 1985), p. 92.

41. Lasch, C. "Why 'the survival mentality' is rife in America." *U.S. News and World Report* (May 17, 1982), p. 59.

42. Rubenstein, C. "Wellness is all: A report on *Psychology Today*'s survey of beliefs about health." *Psychology Today* (October 1982), p. 37.

43. Zola, I. K. "Depictions of disability—metaphor, message, and medium in the media: A research and political agenda." *Social Science Journal* 22 (1985). 1–13.

44. Ibid., pp. 1–13.

45. "Running the Western States 100: The 'desperate dream' of Antonio Rossmann." *Harvard Magazine* (November–December 1985), pp. 84–86.

46. Ibid.

47. Thomas, L. *The Medusa and the Snail*, p. 46.

CHAPTER NINE

1. Harris, L. *Inside America.* (New York: Vintage Press, 1987), p. 41.
2. Shorter, E. *Bedside Manners.* (New York: Simon and Schuster, 1985), pp. 212–214.
3. Ibid., p. 215.
4. Veroff, J., Douvan, E., and Fulka, R. A. *The Inner American.* (New York: Basic Books, 1981), pp. 348–350.
5. Verbrugge, L. M. "Longer life but worsening health? Trends in health and mortality of middle-aged and older persons." *Milbank Memorial Fund Quarterly* 62 (1984): 475–519.
6. Ibid.
7. National Center for Health Statistics. *Selected Health Characteristics by Occupation.* (Washington, DC: USDHEW, DHHS publication #80–1561, Series 10, No. 133, 1980), pp. 11–12.
8. Mishler, E. G., Amarasingham, L. R., Osherson, S. D., et al. *Social Contexts of Health, Illness, and Patient Care.* (New York: Cambridge University Press, 1981).
9. Shorter, E. *Bedside Manners,* pp. 119–120.
10. Freidson, E. *Profession of Medicine.* (New York: Dodd, Mead, 1970), p. 285.
11. Ibid., p. 285.
12. Dubos, R. J. *Mirage of Health.* (New York: Harper and Bros., 1959), p. 22–23.
13. Ibid., see also Dubos, R. J. *Man, Medicine, and Environment.* (London: Pall Mall Press, 1968).
14. Fries, J. F. "Aging, natural death, and the compression of morbidity." *New England Journal of Medicine* 303 (1980): 130–135.
15. Ibid., pp. 130–135.
16. Gruenberg, E. M. "The failures of success." *Milbank Memorial Fund Quarterly* 55 (1977): 3–24.
17. "Erosion of public's confidence in health care system is factor in self-care growth." *Behavioral Medicine Newsletter* 7 (1980): 5.
18. Verbrugge, L. M. "Longer life but worsening health?"
19. Gruenberg, E. M. "The failures of success."
20. Ibid.
21. Fuchs, V. R. *How We Live.* (Cambridge, MA: Harvard University Press, 1983), p. 187.
22. Powles, J. "On the limitations of modern medicine." *Science, Medicine and Man* 1 (1973): 1–30; see also McKeown, T. *The Role of Medicine: Dream, Mirage, or Nemesis.* (Princeton, NJ: Princeton University Press, 1979), pp. 29–78; McDermott, W. "Absence of indicators of the influence of its physicians on a society's health." *American Journal of Medicine* 70 (1981): 833–843.

23. Fuchs, V. R. *Who Shall Live?* (New York: Basic Books, 1974), pp. 9–30; see also Wildavsky, A. "Doing better and feeling worse: The political pathology of health policy." *Daedalus* 106 (1977): 105–123; Maynard, A. "The production of health and health care." *Journal of Economic Studies* 10 (1983): 31–45.

24. Eggertsen, S. C., and Berg, A. O. "Is it good practice to treat patients with uncomplicated myocardial infarction at home?" *Journal of the American Medical Association* 251 (1984): 349–350.

25. Budiansky, S. "A measure of failure." *Atlantic Monthly* (January 1986), p. 32.

26. McKeown, T. *The Role of Medicine: Dream, Mirage, or Nemesis?* (Princeton, NJ: Princeton University Press, 1979).

27. Ibid., pp. 91–113.

28. Steel, K., Gertman, P. M., Crescenzi, C., and Anderson, J. "Iatrogenic illness on a general medical service at a university hospital." *New England Journal of Medicine* 304 (1981): 638–642.

29. Silverman, W. A. "Medical inflation." *Perspectives in Biology and Medicine* 23 (1980): 617–637.

30. Apfel, R. J., and Fisher, S. M. *To Do No Harm: DES and the Dilemmas of Modern Medicine.* (New Haven, CT: Yale University Press, 1984).

31. Ibid., pp. 11–28.

32. Ibid., p. 39.

33. Paffenbarger, R. S., Hyde, R. T., Wing, A. L., Hsieh, C-C. "Physical activity, all-cause mortality, and longevity of college alumni." *New England Journal of Medicine* 314 (1986): 605–613.

34. Fisher, L. M. "A Bandage Boom." *New York Times* (May 24, 1987).

35. Brenton, M. "The Fitness Craze." *Cosmopolitan* (November 1986), p. 277.

36. O'Brien, R. "Rising expectations." *The Runner* (January 1986), p. 56.

37. Toufexis, A. "Watch the bouncing body." *Time* (June 30, 1986), p. 74.

38. Koplan, J. P., Siscovick, D. S., and Goldbaum, G. M. "The risks of exercise: A public health view of injuries and hazards." *Public Health Reports* 100 (1985): 189–195.

39. Yates, A., Leehey, K., and Shisslak, C. M. "Running: An analogue of anorexia?" *New England Journal of Medicine* 308 (1983): 251–255.

40. Ibid.

41. Sheehan, G. "Negative addiction: A runner's perspective." *Physician Sports Medicine* 7 (1979): 49.

42. Associated Press. "Healthy" diet may hinder child's growth, expert says." *Boston Globe* (July 12, 1986).

43. Zaslow, J. "Fourth-Grade Girls These Days Ponder Weighty Matters." *Wall Street Journal* (February 11, 1986).

44. Ibid.

45. Halmi, K. A. "Anorexia Nervosa." In *Comprehensive Textbook of Psychiatry,* 4th edition, ed. H. I. Kaplan and B. J. Sadock. (Baltimore: Williams and Wilkins, 1985), pp. 1143–1148.
46. Ibid., pp. 1143–1148.
47. Wooley, O. W., Wooley, S. "The Beverly Hills eating disorder: The mass marketing of anorexia nervosa." *International Journal of Eating Disorders* 1 (1982): 57–69.
48. Clark, M. "Search for a cure." *Newsweek* (August 7, 1986), p. 61.
49. Winsten, J. A. "Science and the media: The boundaries of truth." *Health Affairs* 4 (1985): 5–23.
50. Goleman, D. "Forgetfulness is seen causing more worry than it should." *New York Times* (July 1, 1986).
51. Phillips, D. P., and Cartensen, L. L. "Clustering of teenage suicides after television news stories about suicide." *New England Journal of Medicine* 315 (1986): 685–689; Gould, M. S. and Shaffer, D. "The impact of suicide in television movies." *New England Journal of Medicine* 315 (1986): 690–694.
52. Weiner, S. L. "Tampons and Toxic Shock Syndrome: Consumer Protection or Public Confusion? In *Consuming Fears: The Politics of Product Risks,* ed. H. M. Sapolsky. (New York: Basic Books, 1986), pp. 141–158.
53. Todd, J. K. "Toxic Shock Syndrome: Scientific uncertainty and the public media." *Pediatrics* 67 (1981): 921–923.
54. Weiner, S. L. "Tampons and Toxic Shock Syndrome."
55. Ibid., pp. 157–158.
56. Brodsky, C. M. " 'Allergic to everything': A medical subculture." *Psychosomatics* 24 (1983): 731–742; Stewart, D. E. "Psychiatric assessment of patients with 20th-century disease ('total allergy syndrome')." *Canadian Medical Association Journal* 133 (1985): 1001–1006; Terr, A. L. "Environmental illness: A clinical review of 50 cases." *Archives of Internal Medicine* 146 (1986): 145–149.
57. Crawford, R. "A Cultural Account of 'Health': Control, Release, and the Social Body." In *Contemporary Issues in Health, Medicine, and Social Policy,* ed. J. B. McKinlay. (New York: Tavistock Publications, 1984), p. 66.
58. Ibid., p. 86.
59. Illich, I. *Medical Nemesis.* (New York: Pantheon Books, 1976), pp. 133–154.
60. Giddon, D. B. "Through the looking glass of physicians, dentists, and patients." *Perspectives in Biology and Medicine* 26 (1983): 451–458.
61. Ibid., pp. 451–458.
62. Freedman, J. L. *Happy People.* (New York: Harcourt Brace Jovanovich, 1978), pp. 131–132.

63. Advertisement for No Nonsense Support Stockings.
64. Prudden, B. *Myotherapy: Bonnie Prudden's Complete Guide to Pain-Free Living.* (New York: Ballantine Books, 1984), dust jacket.
65. Slater, P. *The Pursuit of Loneliness,* 2nd ed. (Boston: Beacon Press, 1976), pp. 138–139.
66. Boffey, P. M. "Thousands in U.S. Receive Treatment in Experiments." *New York Times* (January 1, 1986).

CHAPTER TEN

1. Bakan, D. *Disease, Pain, and Sacrifice.* (Boston: Beacon Press, 1971), pp. 59–67.
2. Ibid., pp. 98–104.
3. Ehrlich, R. *The Healthy Hypochondriac.* (Philadelphia: The Saunders Press, 1980), pp. 10, 54.
4. Slater, P. *The Pursuit of Loneliness.* (Boston: Beacon Press, 1976), pp. 13–18.
5. McCormick, J. S., and Skrabanek, P. "Holy dread." *Lancet* 2 (1984): 1455–1456.
6. Sontag, S. *Illness as Metaphor.* (New York: Vintage Books, 1979), p. 54.
7. Thomas, L. *The Medusa and the Snail.* (New York: Bantam Books, 1979), p. 44.
8. Illich, I. *Medical Nemesis.* (New York: Pantheon Books, 1976), p. 106.
9. Younger, S. J., Allen, M., Bartlett, E. T., et al. "Psychosocial and ethical implications of organ retrieval." *New England Journal of Medicine* 313 (1985): 321–324.
10. Illich, I. *Medical Nemesis,* p. 106.
11. Wallis, C. "To Feed or not to feed?" *Time* (March 31, 1986), p. 60.
12. Younger, S. J., Allen, M., Bartlett, E. T., et al. "Psychosocial and ethical implications of organ retrieval."
13. Ibid., p. 322.
14. Nerem, R. M., Levesque, M. J., and Cornhill, J. F. "Social environment as a factor in diet-induced atherosclerosis." *Science* 208 (1980): 1475–1476.
15. Cabot, R. C., and Dicks, R. L. *The Art of Ministering to the Sick.* (New York: MacMillan, 1936), p. 191.
16. Ibid., p. 193.
17. Kohut, H. *The Restoration of the Self.* (New York: International University Press, 1977).
18. Rako, S., and Mazer, H. *Semrad: The Heart of a Therapist.* (New York: Jason Aronson, 1980), p. 45.
19. Mack, R. M. "Lessons from living with cancer." *New England Journal of Medicine* 311 (1984): 1640–1644.

Index